Anti-Inflammatory Diet for Beginners

4-Week Meal Plan To Heal The Immune System And Activate Your Metabolism. Easy Recipes For Two To Build Your First Line Of Defense Against Chronic Inflammation!

By
Lisa Weil

© Copyright 2021 by Lisa Weil - All rights reserved.

This document is geared towards providing exact and reliable information in regards to the topic and issue covered. The publication is sold with the idea that the publisher is not required to render accounting, officially permitted, or otherwise, qualified services. If advice is necessary, legal or professional, a practiced individual in the profession should be ordered.

- From a Declaration of Principles, which was accepted and approved equally by a Committee of the American Bar Association and a Committee of Publishers and Associations.

In no way is it legal to reproduce, duplicate, or transmit any part of this document in either electronic means or in printed format. Recording of this publication is strictly prohibited, and any storage of this document is not allowed unless with written permission from the publisher. All rights reserved.

The information provided herein is stated to be truthful and consistent, in that any liability, in terms of inattention or otherwise, by any usage or abuse of any policies, processes, or directions contained within is the solitary and utter responsibility of the recipient reader. Under no circumstances will any legal responsibility or blame be held against the publisher for any reparation, damages, or monetary loss due to the information herein, either directly or indirectly.

Respective authors own all copyrights not held by the publisher.

The information herein is offered for informational purposes solely and is universal as such. The presentation of the information is without a contract or any type of guarantee assurance.

The trademarks that are used are without any consent, and the publication of the trademark is without permission or backing by the trademark owner. All trademarks and brands within this book are for clarifying purposes only and are owned by the owners themselves, not affiliated with this document.

Table of Contents

Introduction 11

Chapter 1- Understanding the Concept of Inflammation 12
1.1 What is Inflammation? 12
1.2 Causes of Inflammation 12
1.3 Types of Inflammation 13
1.4 Chronic Inflammatory Diseases 14

Chapter 2-Intestinal Health - An Overview 16
2.1 The 4R Programme 16

Chapter 3- The Anti-Inflammatory Diet 19

Chapter 4- Guide to the Lists of Foods 21
4.1 List of Inflammatory Foods 21
4.2 List of Anti-Inflammatory Foods 29

Chapter 5- Food Shopping List for Anti-Inflammatory Diet 42
5.1 The Anti-Inflammatory Shopping List 42
5.2 Anti-Inflammatory Plate 52
5.3 The Anti-Inflammatory Pantry 53

Chapter 6- 4-Week Meal Plan for an Anti-Inflammatory Diet 55
6.1 Helpful Advises and Suggestions to Get Started 56
6.2 Phase One – The Preparation 56
6.3 Phase Two- The Nourishment and Cleansing 57
6.4 Phase Three- The Reintroduction 58
6.5 Phase Four - Transition to Long-Term Anti-Inflammatory Eating 60
6.6 Meal Plan 61

Chapter 7-Breakfast Recipes 67
7.1 Spinach Frittata 67
7.2 Mushroom and Bell Pepper Omelet 68
7.3 Yogurt, Berry, and Walnut Parfait 68
7.4 Oatmeal and Cinnamon with Dried Cranberries 69
7.5 Green Tea and Ginger Shake 69
7.6 Smoked Salmon Scrambled Eggs 70
7.7 Chia Breakfast Pudding 70
7.8 Coconut Rice with Berries 70
7.9 Overnight Muesli 71

7.10 Spicy Quinoa *72*

7.11 Buckwheat Crêpes with Berries *72*

7.12 Warm Chia-Berry Non-dairy Yogurt *73*

7.13 Buckwheat Waffles *73*

7.14 Coconut Pancakes *74*

7.15 Spinach Muffins *75*

7.16 Herb Scramble with Sautéed Cherry Tomatoes *76*

7.17 Mushroom "Frittata" *76*

7.18 Cucumber and Smoked-Salmon Lettuce Wraps *77*

7.19 Sweet Potato Hash *78*

7.20 Fresh Berry Parfait with Coconut Cashew Cream *78*

7.21 Breakfast Burrito with Chickpeas and Avocado *79*

7.22 Smoked Salmon and Avocado Tartine *79*

7.23 Breakfast Rice with Crumbled Nori *80*

7.24 Sweet Potato Hash with Lamb Sausage *81*

7.25 Sweet or Savory Quinoa Crepes *82*

7.26 Mango Muesli with Brazil Nut Topping *83*

7.27 Power-Packed Granola with Currants and Chia Seeds *83*

Chapter 8-Smoothie Recipes *85*

8.1 Inflammation-Soothing Smoothie *85*

8.2 Kale and Banana Smoothie *85*

8.3 Eat-Your-Vegetables Smoothie *86*

8.4 Cherry Smoothie *86*

8.5 Green Apple Smoothie *87*

8.6 Turmeric and Green Tea Mango Smoothie *87*

8.7 Green Smoothie *88*

8.8 One-for-All Smoothie *88*

8.9 Mango-Thyme Smoothie *89*

8.10 Protein Powerhouse Smoothie *89*

8.11 Chai Smoothie *90*

8.12 Peachy Mint Punch *90*

8.13 Coconut-Ginger Smoothie *91*

8.14 Super Green Smoothie *91*

8.15 Blueberry, Chocolate, and Turmeric Smoothie *92*

8.16 Green Tea and Pear Smoothie *93*

8.17 Ginger-Berry Smoothie *93*

 8.18 Berry Green Power Smoothie 93

Chapter 9-Snacks and Appetizer Recipes..95

 9.1 Cucumber-Yogurt Dip 95

 9.2 White Bean Dip... 95

 9.3 Mashed Avocado with Jicama Slices 96

 9.4 Creamy Broccoli Dip 97

 9.5 Smoked Trout and Mango Wraps 97

 9.6 Kale Chips 98

 9.7 Smoked Turkey–Wrapped Zucchini Sticks 98

 9.8 Crunchy-Spicy Chickpeas 99

 9.9 Sweet Potato Chips 99

 9.10 Mini Snack Muffins 100

 9.11 Strawberry-Chia Ice Pops 101

 9.12 Garlic Ranch Dip 101

 9.13 Blueberry Nut Trail Mix 101

 9.14 Black Bean and Artichoke Hummus 102

 9.15 Crispy Curried Chickpeas 102

 9.16 White Bean and Kalamata Olive Hummus 103

 9.17 Shiitake Mushroom and Walnut Pâté 103

 9.18 Creamy Avocado Spinach Dip 104

 9.19 Artichoke and Basil Tapenade 105

 9.20 Anti-Inflammatory Trail Mix 105

 9.21 Nutty Coconut Energy Truffle 106

 9.22 Tropical Quinoa Power Bars 107

Chapter 10-Lunch Recipes..108

 10.1 Lentils with Tomatoes and Turmeric 108

 10.2 Fried Rice with Kale 109

 10.3 Tofu and Red Pepper Stir-Fry 109

 10.4 Sweet Potato and Bell Pepper Hash with a Fried Egg 110

 10.5 Quinoa Florentine 110

 10.6 Tomato Asparagus Frittata 111

 10.7 Tofu Sloppy Joes 112

 10.8 Broccoli and Egg "Muffins" 112

 10.9 Shrimp Scampi 113

 10.10 Shrimp with Cinnamon Sauce 114

 10.11 Manhattan-Style Salmon Chowder 114

   10.12 Citrus Salmon on a Bed of Greens *115*

   10.13 Salmon Ceviche *116*

   10.14 Rosemary-Lemon Cod *116*

   10.15 Tuscan Chicken *117*

   10.16 Chicken Adobo *117*

   10.17 Chicken Stir-Fry *118*

   10.18 Easy Chicken and Broccoli *118*

   10.19 Chicken Sandwiches with Roasted Red Pepper Aioli *119*

   10.20 Turkey Scaloppine with Rosemary and Lemon Sauce *120*

   10.21 Turkey Burgers with Ginger-Teriyaki Sauce and Pineapple *121*

   10.22 Ground Turkey and Spinach Stir-Fry *121*

   10.23 Pork Chops with Gingered Applesauce *122*

   10.24 Macadamia-Dusted Pork Cutlets *122*

   10.25 Lamb Meatballs with Garlic Aioli *123*

   10.26 Beef Flank Steak Tacos with Guacamole *123*

   10.27 Beef and Broccoli Stir-Fry *124*

   10.28 Beef and Bell Pepper Fajitas *125*

   10.29 Hamburger with Pub Sauce *125*

   10.30 Quinoa-Stuffed Collard Rolls *126*

Chapter 11-Dinner Recipes **128**

   11.1 Whole-Wheat Pasta with Tomato-Basil Sauce *128*

   11.2 Tofu and Spinach Sauté *129*

   11.3 Sweet Potato Curry with Spinach *129*

   11.4 Buckwheat Noodles with Peanut Sauce *130*

   11.5 Kale Frittata *130*

   11.6 Black Bean Chili with Garlic and Tomatoes *131*

   11.7 Mushroom Pesto Burgers *132*

   11.8 Egg Salad Cups *132*

   11.9 Shrimp with Spicy Spinach *133*

   11.10 Pan-Seared Scallops with Lemon-Ginger Vinaigrette *133*

   11.11 Roasted Salmon and Asparagus *134*

   11.12 Orange and Maple-Glazed Salmon *134*

   11.13 Cod with Ginger and Black Beans *135*

   11.14 Halibut Curry *136*

   11.15 Chicken Cacciatore *136*

   11.16 Chicken and Bell Pepper Sauté *137*

11.17 Chicken Salad Sandwiches 137
11.18 Rosemary Chicken 138
11.19 Gingered Turkey Meatballs 138
11.20 Turkey and Kale Sauté 139
11.21 Turkey with Bell Peppers and Rosemary 139
11.22 Mustard and Rosemary Pork Tenderloin 140
11.23 Thin-Cut Pork Chops with Mustardy Kale 141
11.24 Beef Tenderloin with Savory Blueberry Sauce 141
11.25 Ground Beef Chili with Tomatoes 142
11.26 Fish Taco Salad with Strawberry Avocado Salsa 143
11.27 Beef and Bell Pepper Stir-Fry 144
11.28 Veggie Pizza with Cauliflower-Yam Crust 144
11.29 Toasted Pecan Quinoa Burgers 145
11.30 Sizzling Salmon and Quinoa 146

Chapter 12-Soups and Stews Recipes 148

12.1 Roasted Vegetable Soup 148
12.2 Broth Mushrooms 149
12.3 Tomato Soup 149
12.4 Cream of Kale Soup 150
12.5 Squash and Ginger Soup 151
12.6 Easy Summer Gazpacho 151
12.7 Fennel, Leek, and Pear Soup 152
12.8 Pumpkin Soup with Fried Sage 152
12.9 Lentil and Carrot Soup with Ginger 153
12.10 Coconut Curry–Butternut Squash Soup 154
12.11 Soba Noodle Soup with Spinach 155
12.12 Sweet Potato and Rice Soup 155
12.13 Broccoli and Lentil Stew 156
12.14 Winter Squash and Kasha Stew 157
12.15 Chicken Chili with Beans 157
12.16 Mango and Black Bean Stew 158
12.17 Coconut Fish Stew 159
12.18 Gingered Chicken and Vegetable Soup 159
12.19 Curried Sweet Potato Soup 160
12.20 Melon and Green Tea Soup 161
12.21 Beefy Lentil and Tomato Stew 161

12.22 Garlicky Lamb Stew 162

Chapter 13-Sides and salads Recipes 163
13.1 Broccoli-Sesame Stir-Fry 163
13.2 Salmon and Dill Pâté 164
13.3 Chickpea and Garlic Hummus 164
13.4 Citrus Spinach 165
13.5 Brown Rice with Bell Peppers 165
13.6 Guacamole 166
13.7 Spinach and Walnut Salad with Raspberry Vinaigrette 166
13.8 Tomato and Basil Salad 166
13.9 Sautéed Apples and Ginger 167
13.10 Rosemary and Garlic Sweet Potatoes 167
13.11 Mixed Berry Salad with Ginger 168
13.12 Pear-Walnut Salad 168
13.13 Sliced Apple, Beet, and Celery Salad 169
13.14 Avocado and Mango Salad 169
13.15 Almost Caesar Salad 170
13.16 Brussels Sprout Slaw 170
13.17 Vegetable Slaw with Feta Cheese 171
13.18 Mediterranean Chopped Salad 172
13.19 Quinoa and Roasted Asparagus Salad 172
13.20 White Bean and Tuna Salad 173
13.21 Mango Salsa 174
13.22 Roasted Root Vegetables 174
13.23 Turmeric Chicken Salad 175
13.24 Lentil, Vegetable, and Fruit Bowl 176
13.25 Roasted Cauliflower with Almond Sauce 176
13.26 Cauliflower Purée 177
13.27 Green Beans with Crispy Shallots 178
13.28 Roasted Sweet Potatoes and Pineapple 178

Chapter 14-Dessert Recipes 180
14.1 Sweet Spiced Pecans... 180
14.2 Honeyed Apple Cinnamon Compote 181
14.3 Cranberry Compote 181
14.4 Coconut Rice with Blueberries 181
14.5 Greek Yogurt with Blueberries, Nuts, and Honey 182

14.6 Maple-Glazed Pears with Hazelnuts 182
14.7 Green Tea–Poached Pears 183
14.8 Blueberry Ambrosia 183
14.9 Easy Peanut Butter Balls 184
14.10 Chocolate–Almond Butter Mousse 184
14.11 Melon with Berry-Yogurt Sauce 185
14.12 Roasted Peaches with Raspberry Sauce and Coconut Cream 185
14.13 Cherry Ice Cream 186
14.14 Blueberry Crisp 186
14.15 Grilled Pineapple with Chocolate Ganache 187
14.16 Chocolate-Avocado Mousse with Sea Salt 187
14.17 Fruit and Walnut Crumble 188
14.18 Coconut Ice Cream Sandwiches 189
14.19 Chocolate-Cherry Clusters 190
14.20 Gluten-Free Oat and Fruit Bars 191
14.21 Pumpkin Coconut Pie with Almond Crust 191
14.22 Mixed Berry Walnut Crumble 193
14.23 Rustic Pear and Fig Crostatas 193
14.24 So-Easy Coconut Mango Sorbet 194
14.25 Baked Pears or Apples with Cashew Cream 195
14.26 Strawberry Rhubarb Crumble 195
14.27 Vanilla Wafer Pudding 196
14.28 No-Bake Peach Pie 197

Chapter 15-Dressings and Sauces Recipes **198**

15.1 Walnut Pesto 198
15.2 Spinach Pesto 198
15.3 Anti-Inflammatory Mayonnaise 199
15.4 Stir-Fry Sauce 199
15.5 Ginger-Teriyaki Sauce 200
15.6 Garlic Aioli 200
15.7 Raspberry Vinaigrette 201
15.8 Lemon-Ginger Vinaigrette 201
15.9 Peanut Sauce 201
15.10 Garlic Ranch Dressing 202
15.11 Coconut Herb Dressing 202
15.12 Avocado Dressing 203

15.13 Berry Vinaigrette *203*
15.14 Almost Caesar Salad Dressing *204*
15.15 Cherry-Peach Chutney with Mint *204*
15.16 Rosemary-Apricot Marinade *205*
15.17 Green Olive Tapenade *205*
15.18 Kale Pesto *206*
15.19 Honey-Mustard-Sesame Sauce *206*
15.20 Chia Jam *207*
15.21 Slow-Cooker Ghee *207*
15.22 Coconut Cream *208*
15.23 Slow-Cooker Vegetable Broth *208*

Conclusion **209**

Introduction

Inflammation has been the popular talk of the town in health and fitness circles, and it's rapidly establishing a reputation as the root cause of a ton of diseases. With a lot of experience in the nutrition industry, I've seen a variety of diet plans, but I'm not one to hop on the new diet bandwagon. Diet centered on the Mediterranean theme. Diabetes, chronic disease, and cancer are also minimized by eating a Mediterranean diet high in plant-based diets and good fats and oils.

In everyday practice, I see people that are struggling with persistent inflammation-related illnesses. Whatever the case might be, diet may be a powerful treatment for reducing inflammation and restoring body balance. It is my mission to inspire people to cure themselves through food, exercise, sleep, stress control, and mindset. Having even minor dietary modifications may have a significant impact.

Not to mention the fact that is bearing excess fat increases inflammation. So, rather than utilizing calorie-restrictive menus, I literally steer people to foods that help them cope with inflammation, and voila, they start to lose weight. I make choices on which foods to include or remove based on evidence-based nutrition, but I won't bore you with the specifics. This is a really healthy and efficient protocol that involves lots of nutrient-rich foods and a decent mix of protein, fat, and carbohydrates whether you're struggling from chronic inflammation or are attracted to the concept of a "detox" or "cleanse."

This book's meals are perfect for those on a cleanse, as well as anyone on an elimination diet or may have many food allergies. You'll soon realize that this isn't just another diet, but a way of life if you trust yourself to accept the ideas in this book.

Chapter 1- Understanding the Concept of Inflammation

Inflammation is what you've already seen, whether you've ever been hurt or sick. Inflammation is "the body's immune system reaction to a stimulus," according to the US National Library of Medicine. To put it another way, it's what the body does anytime anything potentially dangerous occurs.

The stimulation determines how this happens in the body. If you have a splinter in your finger, for example, the finger can become red and swollen when your body sends inflammatory cells to the region to prevent inflammation and repair the damage. Fever, aches, and pains will arise when foreign bacteria or viruses invade the bloodstream, causing an inflammatory reaction.

1.1 What is Inflammation?

Inflammation is the body's reaction to irritants and pressures from the outer environment. Our wounds cannot cure without inflammation, which is a normal function of our immune response. Chronic inflammation is induced by a number of causes, and when more people become conscious of its consequences, they choose to remove recognized irritants, such as gluten, in order to feel better. Despite the fact that gluten allergy has gained attention, it is not the only irritant that triggers persistent inflammation. Chronic inflammation may cause or exacerbate diseases, including cardiac disease, inflammatory diseases, diabetes, and a variety of other conditions. Chronic inflammation may induce gastrointestinal upset, lethargy, or a general feeling of malaise.

When you're wounded or sick, the immune system responds rapidly, and inflammation plays a significant part in making your body recover. Inflammation can decrease and gradually vanish while you recover. This isn't necessarily the case, though. Chronic inflammation has been a problem for many patients in recent years; something is allowing the inflammation to persist long though the acute period of an accident or infection has passed. Inflammation that persists has no reason and can also be dangerous.

Chronic inflammation has been commonplace in recent decades, and many doctors believe it is at the root of a variety of disorders, including infectious disease, cardiac disease, arthritis, and several others. This movement against diseases dependent on inflammatory responses can be seen in mortality estimates from 1900 to 1997, according to the Autoimmunity Research Foundation. Infectious diseases such as measles, influenza, and diarrhoea were the leading causes of death in 1900, while persistent inflammatory diseases such as a coronary attacks, cancer, and stroke were the leading causes of death in 1997. According to the Foundation, approximately 45 percent of the nation had a persistent inflammatory disorder in 2000, and 21% had several chronic illnesses. These figures are expected to rise steadily until 2030 and beyond. That's a lot of people who are ill.

1.2 Causes of Inflammation

Medical science is trying to figure out what triggers inflammation, and the Autoimmunity Research Foundation says there are many possible causes. Although the data were focused on qualitative experiments that show a connection, it's necessary to remember that correlation does not equate to causation. This implies that, while reasons are suspected, they are not confirmed.

According to the study, there is no definitive proof of a clear connection between triggers and outcomes. This complexity is a part of life.

About the limitations in epidemiological trials, they may also include data for the correct theories centered on broad numbers of people.

The below are several potential triggers of widespread Chronic Inflammation:

1. Abuse and overuse of antibiotics (including in the food supply and through prescribed medications)

2. Dietary considerations (unbalanced essential fatty acids, processed foods, and chemical additives, among others)

3. Environmental considerations (pesticides and endocrine disrupters, among others)

4. Anti-inflammatories, antibacterial chemicals, and other substances (medications) that inhibit immune responses as well as corticosteroids

Other causes that could play a role in chronic inflammation, according to Medical News Today (MNT), include:

1. Autoimmune conditions

2. Obesity is a concern

3. Sleep loss and low sleep quality

1.3 Types of Inflammation

Three are major two types of inflammation: -

- Acute inflammation
- Chronic inflammation

Acute Inflammation

Acute or short-term inflammation may occur as a result of an accident or illness.

Acute inflammation manifests itself in five ways:

1. Pain can be present all of the time or sometimes when an individual reaches the infected region.

2. The blood flow to the capillaries in the region has increased, resulting in redness.

3. You might have trouble rotating a joint, breathing, smelling, and so on.

4. If fluid builds up in the body, a disease known as edema may occur.

5. Because of the increased blood supply, the affected region can feel warm to the touch.

These indicators do not often appear. Inflammation may be "silent," causing no effects. An individual can also experience fatigue, general malaise, and a fever.

Acute inflammatory symptoms last a few days. The period of subacute inflammation is 2–6 weeks.

Acute inflammation can result from any one of the following: -

1. An injury

2. Exposure to a substance, such as a bee sting or dust

3. An infection

Acute bronchitis, appendicitis, and other diseases resulting in "-itis" may cause acute inflammation, as can an ingrown toenail, a sore throat from a cold or flu, and physical damage or fracture.

Chronic Inflammation

Chronic inflammation may occur if an individual has one or more of the following conditions:

1. Anytime the body detects anything it shouldn't, inflammation occurs. An allergy may develop as a consequence of hypersensitivity to an external stimulus.

2. Chronic inflammation may result from long-term, low-level exposure to an irritant, such as an industrial chemical.

3. Psoriasis is an example of an autoimmune disease in which the immune system incorrectly destroys normal healthy tissue.

4. Autoinflammatory disorders, such as Behçet's disease, are caused by a genetic mechanism that influences the immune system's function.

5. An individual cannot completely recover from acute inflammation in certain instances. This may also result in persistent inflammation.

1.4 Chronic Inflammatory Diseases

CIDs are a form of inflammatory disease.

A host of illnesses have been related to persistent inflammation as the study progresses. The following is a list of several of them.

However, the document is too lengthy to include any of the diseases.

Autoinflammatory Disease

The autoinflammatory disorder is a comparatively recent form that is separate from autoimmune disease, according to the National Institutes of Health's (NIH) National Institution of Arthritis and Musculoskeletal and Skin Disorders (NIAMS).

There are a lot of similarities between the titles, and they do have the same features. Autoimmune conditions are caused by the immune system targeting and inflaming sensitive tissue. The process underlying this response is unclear.

Autoinflammatory disorders are characterized by cycles of severe, recurrent inflammation, which can result in symptoms such as fever and joint pain, and joint swelling.

The following diseases are among them:

- Chronic Atypical Neutrophilic Dermatosis with Lipodystrophy and Elevated Temperature (CANDLE)
- Familial Mediterranean Fever (FMF)
- Tumour Necrosis Factor Receptor-Associated Periodic Syndrome (TRAP)
- Bechet's disease
- Deficiency of the Interleuken-1 Receptor Agonist (DIRA)
- Neonatal Onset Multisystem Inflammatory Disease (NOMID)

Autoimmune Disease

A chronic inflammatory portion is also present in autoimmune disorders, according to NIAMS. Your body destroys healthy tissue as it views it as a hostile invader. Inflammation is one of the most common symptoms of autoimmune disorder, though other symptoms can also be present based on the disease.

According to the American Autoimmune Related Diseases Association (AARDA), there are more than 80 autoimmune diseases actually known. There are many too many to mention here, but here are a couple of the more prevalent autoimmune diseases:

- Ankylosing spondylitis
- Crohn's disease
- Fibromyalgia
- Hashimoto's disease
- Juvenile arthritis
- Lupus
- Multiple sclerosis
- Rheumatoid arthritis
- Addison's disease
- Celiac disease
- Endometriosis
- Grave's disease
- Interstitial cystitis
- Juvenile (type 1) diabetes
- Lyme disease (chronic)
- Psoriasis
- Scleroderma
- Vitiligo
- Ulcerative colitis

Cardiovascular Diseases

Although it is not yet known that inflammation is the cause of cardiovascular disease (heart and blood vessel diseases), the American Heart Association states that it is usually present, especially in the arteries of people who have this illness.

Many conditions related to heart disease, such as smoking, elevated blood pressure, and high levels of "bad" cholesterol known as low-density lipoprotein (LDL), induce inflammation, so lowering these risk factors is vital for disease prevention.

Obesity and Type 2 Diabetes

A study published in the Journal of Clinical Investigation on May 2, 2005, looked into the relationship between type 2 (adult-onset) diabetes, inflammation, and stress and discovered a strong association between inflammation and type 2 diabetes, which was primarily due to obesity. Obesity, according to this line of study, sets off a chain of chemical reactions in the body that trigger systemic inflammation, which contributes to metabolic diseases, including type 2 diabetes.

Chapter 2-Intestinal Health - An Overview

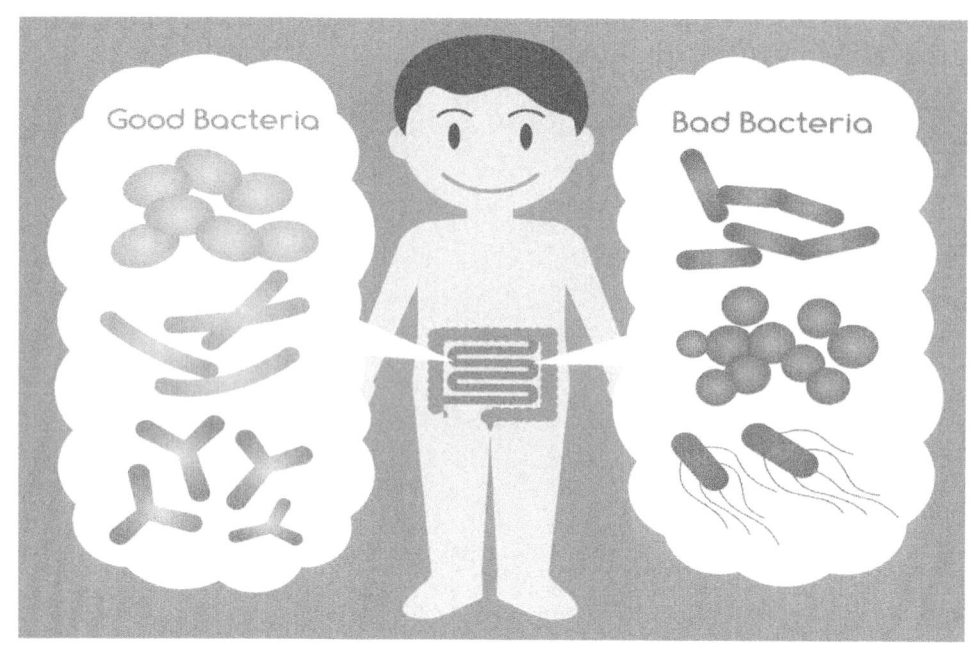

The intestinal system is crucial to good health. Since the lining of the gastro-intestine is constantly subjected to a number of toxins, microbes, and nutrients from the food and water we eat on a daily basis, the digestive tract is easily accessible by the outside environment.

As a result, you will appreciate the significance of preserving healthy gut fitness. Microorganisms in our tract of gastro-intestine have been shown to affect not just our capacity to ingest and consume food efficiently and control bowel activity but also other processes such as the immune system's growth and function, the body's inflammatory and oxidative pathways as well as the vascular system.

Bad gut health, it points out, has an effect on almost every body-organ, bodily function, and illness, whereas improved gut health, will significantly increase autoimmune diseases, diabetes, chronic back pain, obesity, and migraines.

While some traditional practitioners may dismiss these improvements as unrelated or accidental cures, more are integrating this approach into their patient treatment.

Consult the healthcare provider to decide what you should be watching and tracking, may screening testing you might consider, and any short-term changes you should create. Inquire for reputable outlets of recent results that are important to your individual variables. Create a timetable for investigation and evaluation. Determine the treatment's short- and long-term objectives. If you don't have access to a healthcare facility, you should follow a quadratic-step plan to determine possible causes and behaviors that can intensify, prolong, or change how you feel.

2.1 The 4R Programme

The 4R Programme is a screening and guidance service that will help the overwhelming number of chronic condition patients.

It is a variation of the naturopathic technique known as the 3R method, which is derived from a program initially created by Jeffrey Bland, Ph.D., at the Institute for Functional Medicine. Each "R" represents a phase in the procedure.

1. Remove

Remove any ingredients that might produce contaminants from your diets, such as high-heavy-metal-content nutritional supplements, seafood from proven or possibly contaminated streams, and corn-fed beef raised on antibiotics and growth hormones. Remove any foods that cause the body to respond negatively—that is, any foods that you notice don't agree with you. This includes items to which you seem to be allergic. Delete dairy from your diet if you have lactose intolerance symptoms and wheat from your diet if you have gluten intolerance symptoms.

Remove all items that contain added (non-natural) sugar, artificial colors, or preservatives.

Coffee, nicotine and nonsteroidal anti-inflammatory drugs are also irritants to the intestinal lining. Restoring the normal equilibrium of the intestinal flora is critical as it becomes unbalanced, which may impair nutrient absorption and induce chronic low-grade inflammation. There are a variety of reasons for this type of imbalance, which may vary from moderate to extreme. Similarly, signs may range from moderate gastrointestinal (GI) upset to extreme malabsorption, which may necessitate hospitalization.

2. Replace and the supplement

Another "R" in the 4R stands for "The Replace and Supplement," and it applies to those who are unable to produce digestive enzymes. As the name implies, pancreatic insufficiency causes an unwillingness to ingest food and consume nutrients, as well as gas, bloating, and general abdominal pain. Digestion enzyme substitutes or herbal bitters, or the betaine-Houttuynia-cordata injections (HCl) can help stimulate stomach acids.

3. Re-inoculate and re-establish

The next step is to rebalance the microbiota in the intestines such that beneficial bacteria outnumber harmful bacteria. Replace the innocuous bacteria steadily to prevent gas production and intestinal cramping. Start with three billion CFU of the healthy bacterias (bifidobacteria and lactobacillus species) or the yeast (saccharomyces boulardii) per day. Foods have the potential to be the main source of nutrition.

Look for items that have the "Live & Active Cultures" seal, which was developed by the National Yogurt Association, the industry's charitable trade organization in the US. According to the seal, a frozen product must contain at least ten million cultures per gram, whereas a refrigerated commodity must contain at least a hundred million cultures per gram. Read the label before you shop and make sure there's a lot more than the absolute minimum.

Kefir, which includes a wide variety of microbes, including yeast and bacteria, is another source. Lactose-intolerant people can tolerate kefir because it goes through a fermentation process that has just a small amount of lactose. Kimchi and sauerkraut are both good references. These foods are thought to inoculate the intestine with beneficial bacteria and help in improving the health and number of beneficial bacteria on days that you need to supplement your whole-food consumption to achieve your CFU targets.

You will see positive changes in your bowel frequency, bowel consistency, and bowel symptoms when you get significant types and quantities of healthy microflora from your diets or dietary supplements. Go for your gut feeling, despite what the label says!

4. Repair (Intestinal lining)

After two or three weeks of reinoculation, it's time to patch the gut lining. For at least three months, take one to three grams of fish oil, ten milligrams of zinc, six grams of each of the l-glutamine and amino acids glycine, and one gram of pantothenic acid. The gut's inner lining will be effectively rebuilt, enabling it to absorb and digest nutrients while reducing the intake of foreign or toxic compounds that cause inflammation.

We'll go to the pantry and look at the foods that are most necessary for improvement, with that in mind in chapters to come next.

Chapter 3- The Anti-Inflammatory Diet

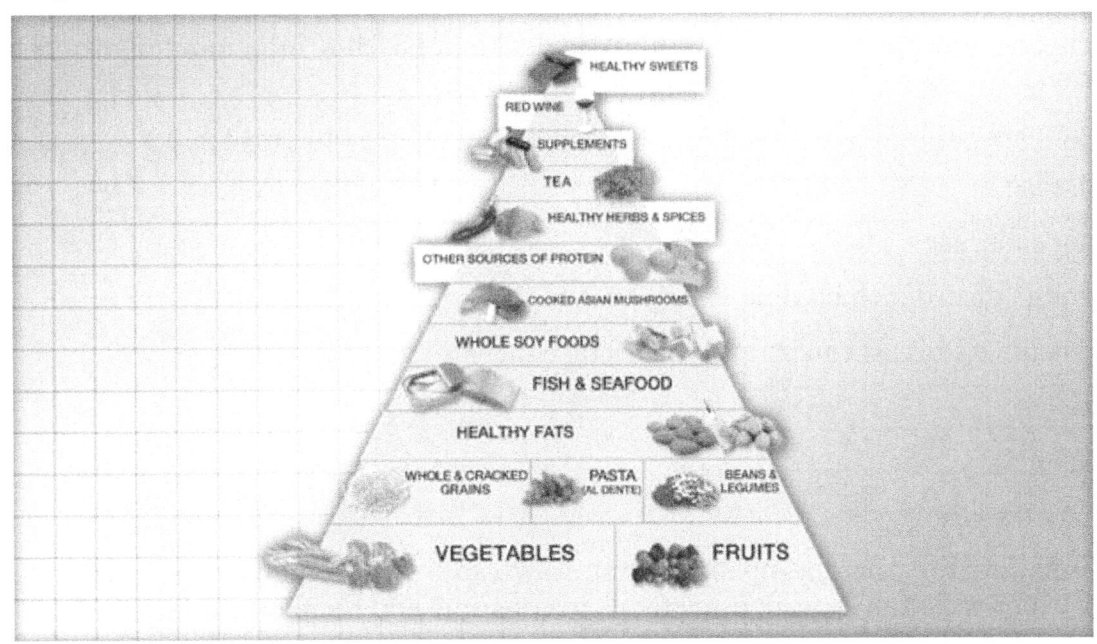

The anti-inflammatory diet is a relatively recent idea that is still being researched. An anti-inflammatory eating pattern close to the Mediterranean diet, which matches the ratio of essential fatty acids (omega-3 to omega-6 fatty acids) and consists mainly of fresh fruits, vegetables, legumes, and whole grains while minimizing saturated fats (such as fats from meat) and optimizing monounsaturated fats, was reported in a study published in the December 2010 issue of Nutrition in Clinical Practice.

Although the recipes and treatments in this book are a helpful place to start, it's still crucial to speak with your primary healthcare physician regarding specific anti-inflammatory techniques. Never use over-the-counter NSAIDs to self-medicate systemic inflammation for longer than a day or two owing to the unintended side effects. Instead, see a doctor or another competent healthcare professional to assess the suitable medical options.

There isn't a formal diet schedule that specifies what to consume, how much to eat, and what to eat. Instead, the anti-inflammatory diet focuses on using foods that have been shown to reduce inflammation while also excluding foods that have been shown to add to it.

Think about the anti-inflammatory diet as a lifestyle rather than a diet, says Brittany Scanniello, RD, a nutritionist in Boulder, Colorado. "An anti-inflammatory diet is a way of living that aims to suppress or prevent low-grade inflammation in our bodies," she explains.

In an ideal world, you'd consume eight or nine servings of fruits and vegetables a day, reduce red meat and dairy consumption, choose complex carbohydrates over simple carbohydrates, and avoid refined foods.

Foods high in omega-3 fatty acids, such as anchovies, tuna, halibut, and mussels, are preferable to omega-6 fatty acids, which can be contained in corn oil, mayonnaise, vegetable oil, salad dressings, and certain refined foods.

Scanniello believes that living this way is beneficial to everyone because all of the ingredients that can induce inflammation are unhealthy in the first place. "I agree that reducing or removing sugar and heavily refined ingredients in favor of unsaturated fats, vegetables, fruits, seeds, nuts, and lean proteins will help everyone," says Scanniello.

She believes that an anti-inflammatory diet may be particularly beneficial for people who suffer from persistent inflammation as a consequence of a medical condition. Athletes and people who engage in high-intensity exercise and want to reduce their baseline inflammation can benefit from this; she says.

Following an anti-inflammatory diet has been shown to help people with:

- Heart disease
- Alzheimer's disease
- Autoimmune disorders including **RA** and MS
- Cancer, including breast cancer and colorectal cancer
- Diabetes
- Epilepsy
- Pulmonary disease

The anti-inflammatory diet has no significant drawbacks, but there might be a learning curve to mastering which inflammation-fighting foods to consume and the foods to resist.

If your daily diet is heavy on refined foods, meat, and dairy, you may need some time to adapt. You'll want to get rid of any highly inflammatory ingredients from your fridge and pantry, and you'll also need to spend some time and money meal prepping because fast food isn't allowed in this diet.

Chapter 4- Guide to the Lists of Foods

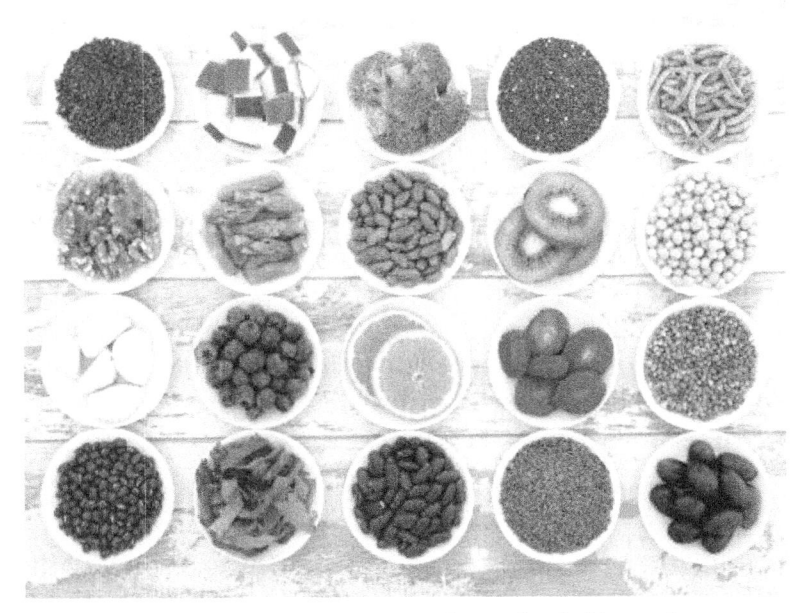

Various dietary methods to treating my symptoms have had direct impacts on me over my life. I felt sluggish when I consumed fast food. I felt tired when I consumed a ton of sugar. My body let me know when I consumed foods that didn't fit along with my body's needs. I feel good and healthy when I consumed balanced foods that helped my fitness. There was definitely a link between what I consumed and how I thought. With that in mind, I'll go through the fundamentals of a dietary solution to persistent inflammatory treatment.

4.1 List of Inflammatory Foods

Here under are provided primary inflammatory foods that are to be avoided in order to follow the diet and are also injurious to our health.

Alcohol

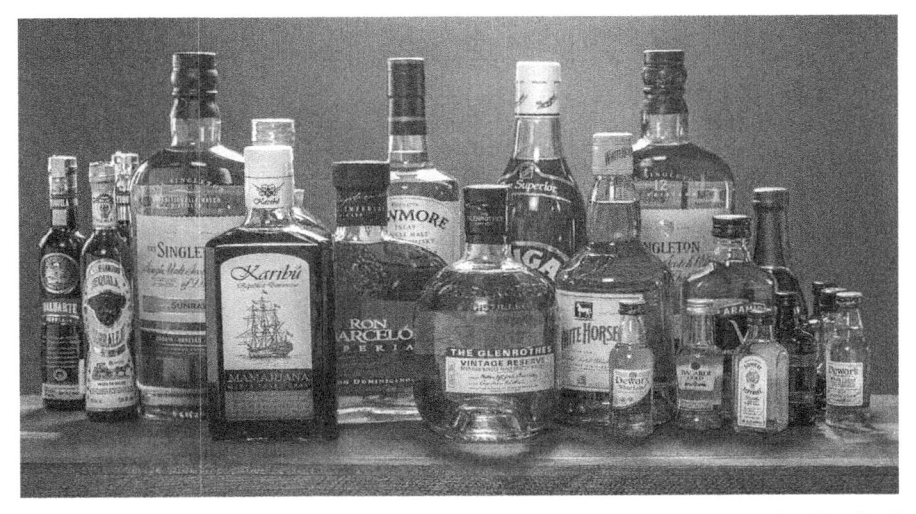

If you want to reduce inflammation, you'll need to figure out how much alcohol you can handle and which kinds are the safest. In small doses, alcohol increases the healthy cholesterol (HDL), decreases insulin regulation, and inhibits blood clotting. Adults who consume moderate amounts of alcohol most days of the week are 25 to 40% less likely to have heart problems and strokes than someone who drinks too frequently or none at all, according to research.

How much is sufficient? Women should drink one serving and men one or two servings on most days of the week, according to studies. 5 oz [150 ml] champagne, 12 oz [360 ml] malt, and 112 oz [45 ml] hard liquor constitute one meal. Women can consume fewer than men since larger amounts deplete folic acid, which triggers a slew of issues, including a 40% increase in the incidence of breast cancer.

For certain people, alcohol may be troublesome. Many East Asians, for example, have a genetic variant that causes them to emit more acetaldehyde after drinking alcohol than other cultures. Acetaldehyde is a poisonous substance that induces nausea, headaches, and flushing of the eyes. If you drink and have this reaction, you're six to ten times more likely to have oesophageal cancer. If you're gluten-intolerant, you'll want to drink gluten-free beer, so many breweries are made from gluten-containing grains like wheat, barley, or rye. Interestingly, the distillation procedure used to manufacture hard liquor eliminates gluten, so gluten-intolerant individuals will sometimes consume rye whiskey, for example. People with celiac disease, on the other hand, have been recorded to have negative responses to hard liquor.

It's more definitely because of the tannin level in red wine that you get headaches after consuming it. Tannins are responsible for the astringent flavor (that harsh, puckering sensation) found in particular wines. According to a new report, people who drank red wines with lower tannin content had fewer headaches than those who drank red wines with higher tannin content. Do your homework and look for wines with lower tannin levels. Cabernet Sauvignon and Merlot from South America have fewer tannins than Malbec from the same area, as well as fewer tannins than their French counterparts.

Limiting the consumption of sugar and processed carbs, as well as your preference for alcohol, is a vital aspect of an anti-inflammatory diet. Liquor is highly distilled and therefore sugar-free; nevertheless, the sugar content of anything you add to the drink can differ significantly. The sugar and carbohydrate level of "light" and pilsner beers, as well as dry wines, is smaller than that of their equivalents.

Corn

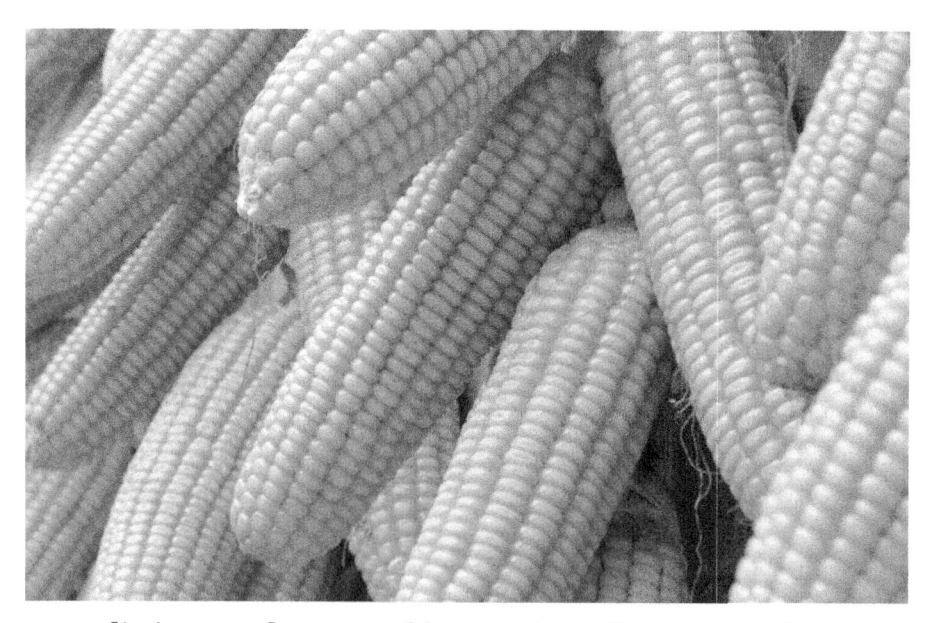

Corn has become my diet's second most problematic ingredient. When I discovered I was gluten intolerant, I began substituting corn for flour in tortillas, wraps, and even some kinds of pasta. When I ate a tonne of corn, though, I also had abdominal discomfort.

What I went through was a textbook case of immune-response cross-reactivity. Antibodies to some gluten proteins had formed in me, and these antibodies could react with proteins from other food groups, like corn. When I consume corn, my immune system recognizes it as a foreign invader and produces antibodies to combat it, causing body aches and a variety of other symptoms. I found that being on a complete deprivation diet can be highly beneficial. When I reintroduced corn to my diet, my symptoms increased, proving that corn is a cause of food for me.

Even if you like corn and your immune system doesn't object to it, keep in mind that in 2012, genetically engineered sweet corn was introduced into the US. Corn is extensively treated with pesticides during harvest, so opting for organic is the healthier option. Still buy registered organic corn to prevent consuming GMO corn and being exposed to toxic pesticides and herbicides. More details about this subject can be found at the Non-GMO Project, an organization dedicated to non-GMO food education and restoration.

Food coloring

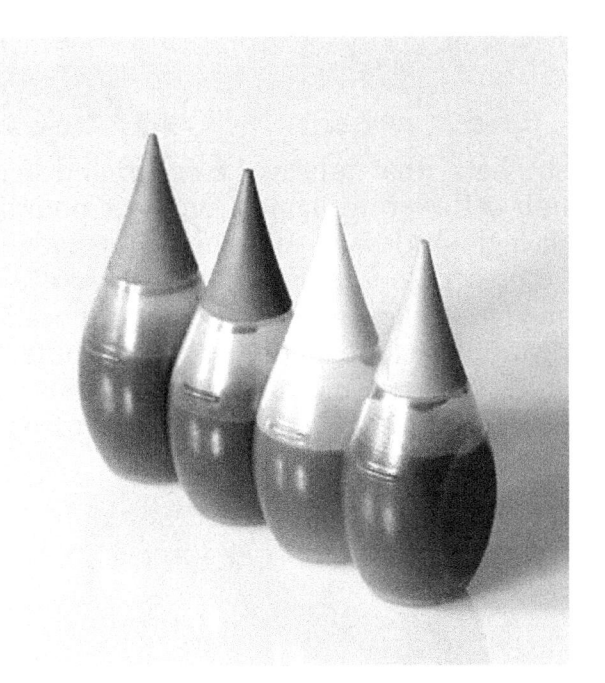

Children's personality changes, such as hyperactivity, anger, frustration, and irritability, have been linked to artificial food coloring. Since the 1950s, our everyday use of artificial food coloring has risen fivefold, as determined by the amount of dye approved by the US Food and Drug Administration for use in consumables. FD&C Green No. 3, Red No. 3 and 40, and Blue No. 1 and 2 are examples of these additives. Although we do recognize that the additives in chemical food coloring are harmful to our health, no one has ever measured how much we consume. In the 1970s, studies assumed that children consumed 20 to 30 mg of artificial coloring every day and used this theory to assess the safety of food coloring. Children are eating far larger doses of food coloring than historically thought, according to a 2014 Purdue University report that measured the precise quantities of different consumer goods. These artificial additives were commonly used in 35 mg per serving in cereals, drinks, and candy. Kids, as you would expect, might comfortably surpass a regular dosage of 100 mg, which is more than three times the dose previously studied. Look for natural food colorings created from beets, saffron, elderberry, turmeric, paprika, and butterfly pea if you choose to use it.

Nightshades

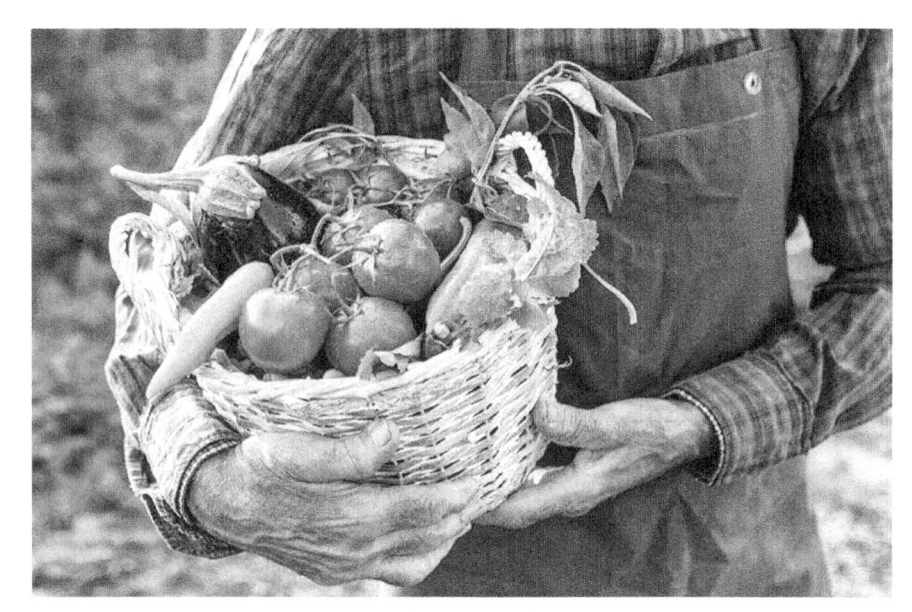

The green elfish "hats" that attach the fruits and vegetables to their stems distinguish the Nightshades family of flowering plants. Eggplants, potatoes, bell peppers, chiles, and tomatoes are the most popular nightshades we eat. Many nightshades provide beneficial nutrients, such as the vitamins A and C present in tomatoes, as well as several antioxidants. Nightshades, on the other hand, are high in glycoalkaloids, which are natural pesticides that may exacerbate joint pain and other arthritic symptoms (and potentially contribute to leaky gut.) What's the bottom line? Eggplants, potatoes, peppers, and tomatoes, whether you're not allergic to nightshades, will be delicious additions to your diet. In this book, I've mentioned alternate ingredients when they're required, just in case you're allergic.

Sugar

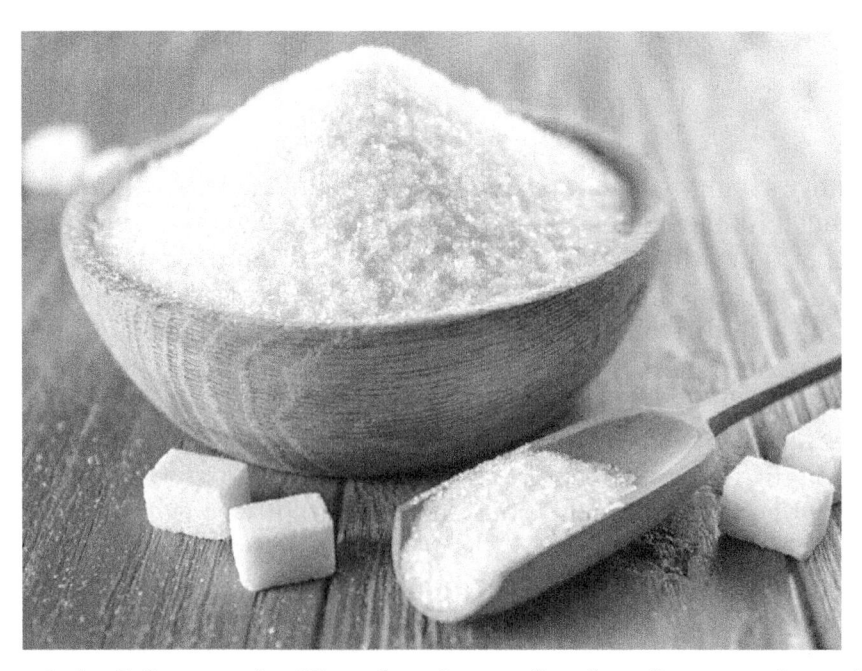

We all know sugar is bad for us, significantly when refined and contaminated with pesticides. However, we live in a natural environment where sugar is present in almost everything, so use it sparingly. (I do use refined sugar now and then to create a traditional cake for special occasions.)

Sugar is the most common food additive in our diet. Sugar is added to almost everything, and it's mostly covered. Spaghetti sauce, crackers, hot dogs, cereals, peanut butter, pizza, canned rice, yogurt, luncheon meats, among other foods, include it. Added sugars are labeled as "brown sugar," "corn syrup," "corn sweetener," "fruit juice concentrates," "honey," "invert sugar," "high fructose corn syrup," "malt sugar," "raw sugar," "molasses," "sugar," "syrup," and "simple syrup" on product labels. Look for terms like sucrose, dextrose, lactose, glucose, and maltose that end in "ose."

Sugar, including sex and addictive substances, fills the gratification region of our brain, known as the nucleus accumbens, with dopamine, according to studies. Manufacturers substituted calories obtained from fat with added sugar as low-fat diets were introduced in the 1980s. Between 1950 and 2000, average sugar intake rose by 40%, from 110 to 152 lb [50 to 69 kg] per year, thanks to the invention of high-fructose corn syrup. This amounts to 32 teaspoons [160 grams] of sugar consumed every day; it's no wonder, then, that rates of prediabetes and diabetes among teens have risen from 9% to 23% between 2000 and 2008. Sugar intake can be limited to 10 teaspoons [40 g] a day, which is the equivalent of consuming a 12-ounce [260-ml] soft drink. This added sugar has a significant impact. Drinking one can of soda a day, for example, raises a child's risk of being obese by 60% and an adult's risk of becoming type 2 diabetic by 80%.

Remember that processed carbohydrates, including white flour, are rapidly transformed into sugar molecules throughout the body and are therefore the same as consuming sugar in its natural state. Calories from added sugar or processed carbs have a powerful, harmful impact on the body, leaving you to crave delicious snacks only a few hours after feeding. Calories from fat and protein, on the other side, keep you happier and fuller for longer, reducing sugar cravings.

Coffee

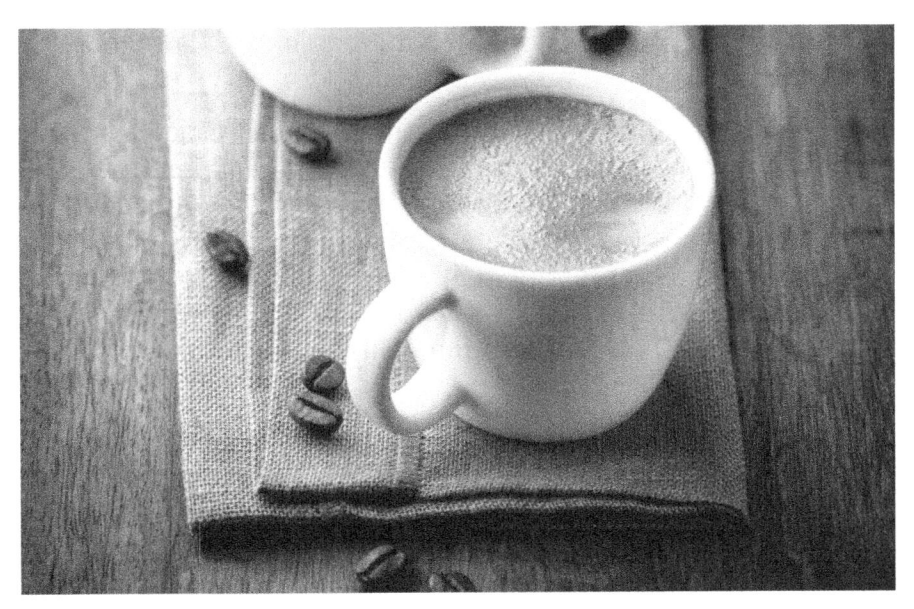

Coffee's antioxidant properties are well established, and consuming 2 to 3 cups (12 to 18 oz [320 to 530 ml]) a day boosts cardiovascular function while drinking more is dangerous. Some people have stomach upset from coffee's tannins, which irritate the stomach lining and aggravate gastroesophageal reflux. Coffee can be avoided if the blood pressure is too high. Caffeinated coffees activate the sympathetic nervous system's "fight or flee" stress reflex, which may lead to increased anxiety, irritability, and irritation, as well as poor sleep.

Dairy

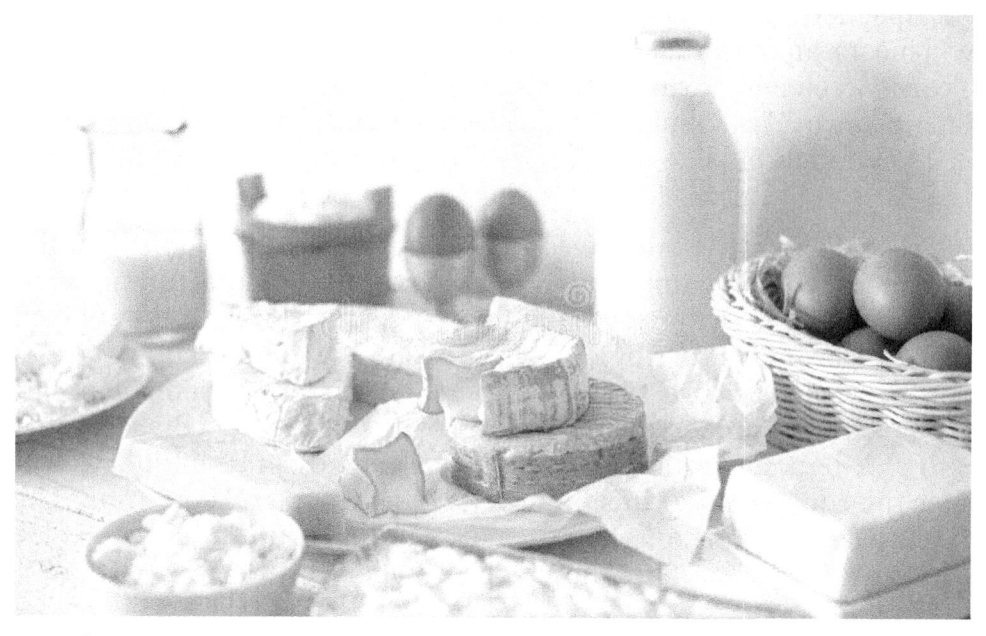

Lactose allergy and casein sensitivity are the two most common forms of dairy intolerance. Lactose sensitivity is a condition in which the lactose sugar in dairy products is unable to be digested. African Americans, Latinos, and Asians, as well as around 20% of Caucasians, are affected by this digestive problem. Within hours after consuming dairy, typical signs include significant discomfort, abdominal bloating and discomfort, and diarrhea. Lactose is used of the highest concentrations in milk and ice cream, causing the most effects. While the amounts in yogurt are close, the live cultures in yogurt seem to render it a more tolerable dairy food for people with this disorder.

Casein allergy is comparable to gluten sensitivity in that the body produces antibodies against the main protein ingredient of the meal, in this case, casein. As a result, patients who are sensitive to casein have gastrointestinal and extra-gastrointestinal effects comparable to those who are sensitive to gluten. Those that are gluten intolerant and others that are casein intolerant have a lot in common. With the potential exception of yogurt, all healing systems believe the dairy goods cause mucus and inflammation in the body. If you have persistent sinusitis, environmental allergies, headaches, or excessive mucus formation, you may want to try cutting out dairy for four weeks to see how you feel.

If you think that cutting out dairy helps your fitness, you'll need to find other calcium sources. Adults require 700 mg of calcium a day, according to new studies, but higher levels are linked to an elevated risk of heart disease and a slight decrease in osteoporosis or hip fractures. Broccoli rabe, soy beans, bok choy, collard greens, and salmon and canned sardines are also good non-dairy calcium sources (with bones). Almond and orange juice, rice milk, and tofu are all fortified sources.

Gluten

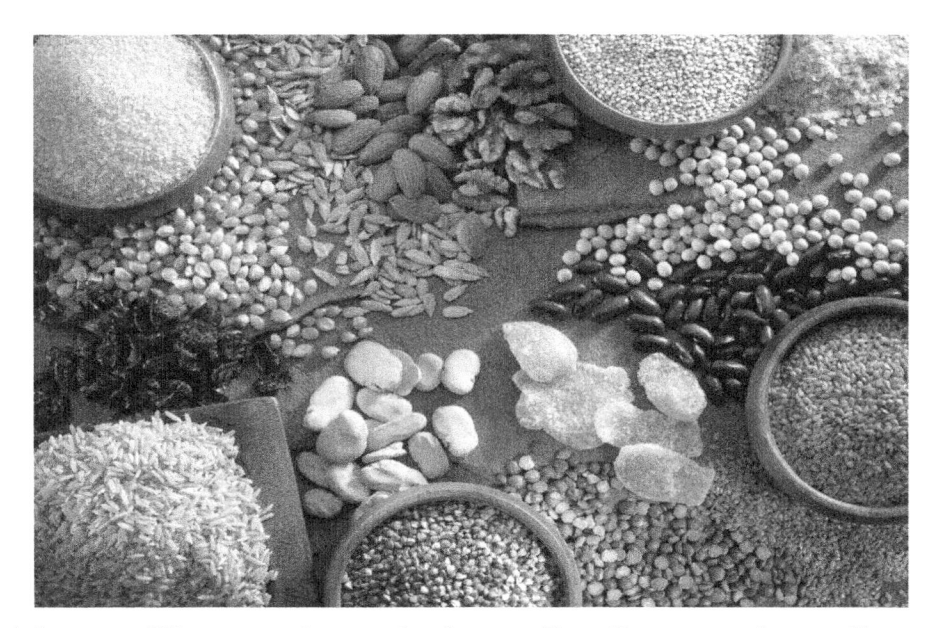

If you're one of the 24 million Americans who have celiac disease or gluten allergy, you can avoid gluten-containing grains like barley, wheat, rye, and oats.

Celiac disease patients have a form of adaptive immune response that is unique to one or more gluten proteins. When antibodies come into contact with gluten proteins, a robust inflammatory response develops, causing intestinal lining damage (also known as "leaky gut"). Gluten and other proteins, as well as pathogens and microbes, are then enabled to pass across the gut-blood membrane, resulting in irritation and extra-gastrointestinal symptoms, including nausea, joint aches, and headaches. Celiac syndrome is diagnosed by specific laboratory tests which have hereditary and family determinants.

Gluten allergy in those who aren't celiac remains a mystery. It is thought to be a milder response than celiac disease. Since people's immune responses are generally nonspecific, others do not produce gluten-specific antibodies. Following the consumption of these ingredients, these people typically feel less inflammation of the gut lining. These patients, on the other hand, have signs that are close to celiac disease, such as bloating, gas, and discomfort, as well as extra-gastrointestinal symptoms.

Skin prick checks, wheat Ig-E blood tests, and a diet challenge will all be used to detect wheat allergy. If you're concerned about a gluten-related condition, follow an abstinence plan for four weeks and still keeping a log of the symptoms. Get screened for wheat allergy and celiac disease if you feel stronger. If all checks come out negative, you most definitely have a nonceliac gluten allergy or something called FODMAPs, which was discovered in the late 1990s by Dr. Sue Shepard.

"Fermentable oligo-, di-, mono-, and polysaccharides and polyols" is the acronym for "fermentable oligo-, di-, mono-, and polysaccharides. Since people with this disorder have trouble swallowing this group of short-chain carbohydrates, physicians warn them to avoid foods like ice cream, ricotta cheese, cashews, lentils, miso, gluten, strawberries, blackberries, artichokes, and cauliflower, which include lactose, fructose, fructans, sugar alcohols, and Galatians. Sufferer's experience feeling much healthier after avoiding certain ingredients for one or two weeks.

In baking and frying, a variety of grains and healthy natural flours may be substituted for standard wheat flour. The secret, just as with refined wheat flours, is restraint.

Here's where I go when I need to duplicate gluten: I use rice flour, almond flour, chickpea flour, buckwheat, and mixes of both of these as wheat-flour substitutes. I use one of the flours made to behave as closely as possible to white flour in baking, such as Cup4Cup or Bob's Red Mill Gluten-Free Flour Mix, for wheat-flour alternatives.

Sugar Substitutes

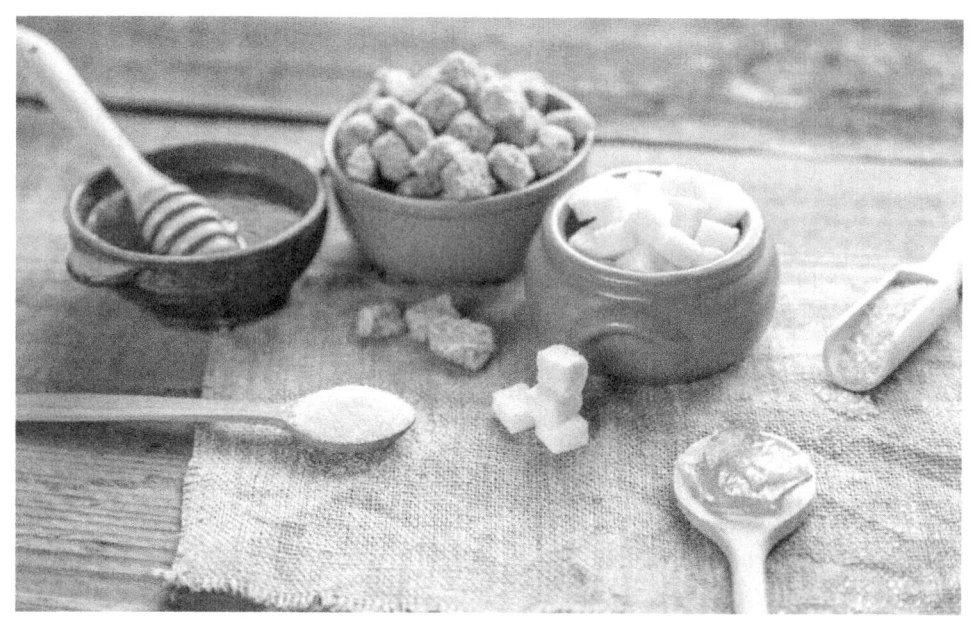

The dangers and benefits of sugar substitutes like aspartame (Equal), sucralose (Splenda), and saccharin (Sweet N Low) have only been studied in a small number of studies. However, a new study reported in the scientific research journal "Nature" discovered that sugar replacements would significantly impair our bodies' capacity to absorb sugar, even as opposed to sugar consumption. The researchers found that noncaloric artificial sweeteners (NAS) affect the microbiota in the gastrointestinal tract in a way that alters how the body absorbs glucose (sugar), leading to a disease known as glucose sensitivity (also known as insulin resistance), which leads to diabetes.

According to the new study, we can stop NAS at all costs. If you just want to boost the flavor, use a small amount of added sugar instead.

Salt

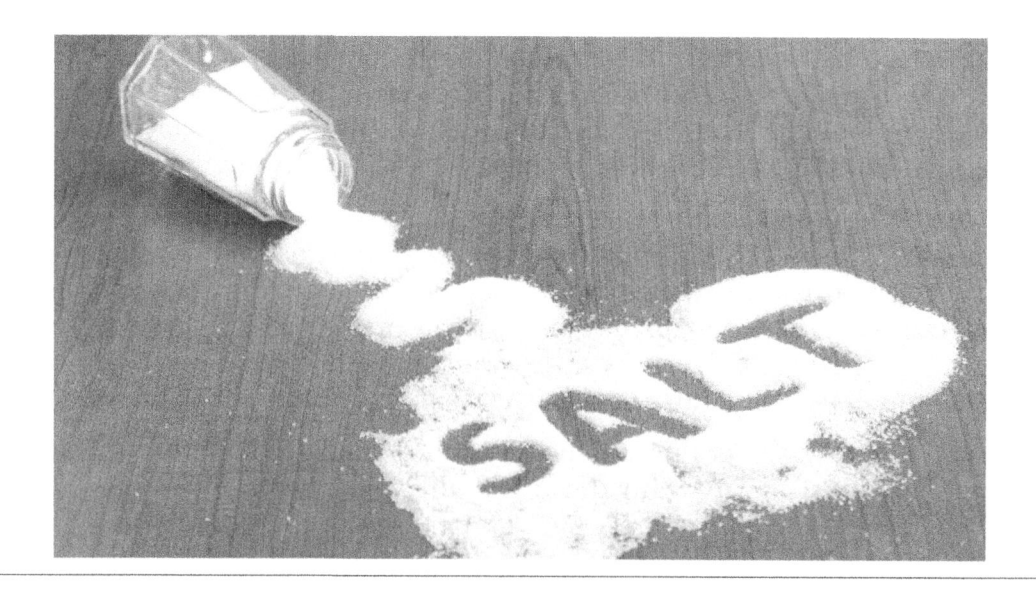

Have you ever found that what one individual deems to be excessively salted, another deems to be insufficiently salted? Your sense of saltiness is influenced by how much salt you've had recently. Since your taste buds adapt quickly, you won't feel a change in the saltiness of your food after seven days if you will find your salt consumption. High blood pressure and kidney failure may be caused by eating so much salt. People over 50 or with elevated blood pressure can consume less than 2,400 mg sodium (1 teaspoon table salt) a day, and preferably less than 1,500 mg.

Since salt is about 40% sodium by weight, 1,500 mg sodium a day equals about 4,000 mg salt. Preparing your own recipes, enhancing flavors, and avoiding frozen, dried, and fast snacks are the easiest ways to skip the salt.

4.2 List of Anti-Inflammatory Foods

Here under is provided the list of critical anti-inflammatory foods that are to be consumed while on the anti-inflammatory diet.

Animal proteins: grass-fed organic chicken, pork, lamb, and beef

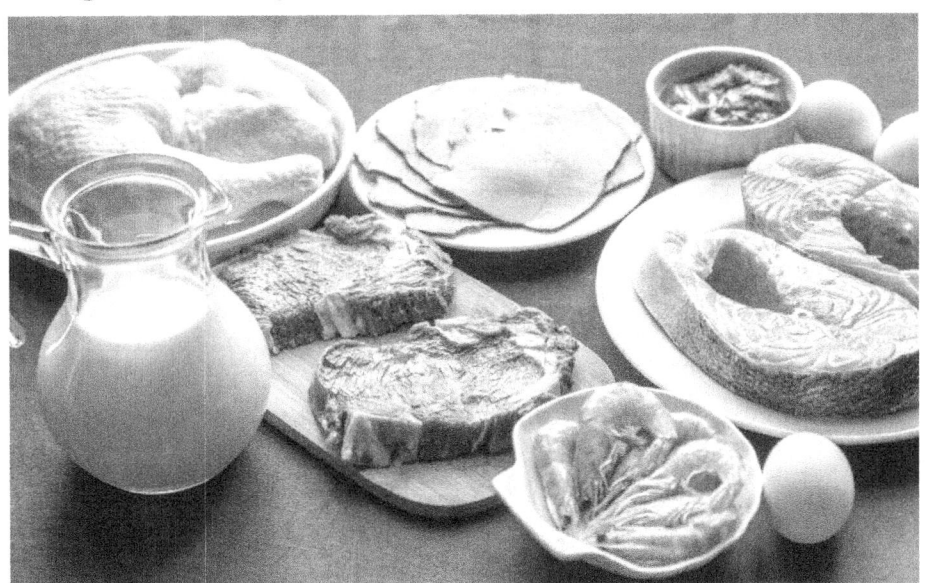

Organic and grass-fed free-range animals are healthier, and their meat is more nutritious and less harmful than meat from conventionally raised livestock. When opposed to corn-fed livestock, pasture-raised poultry, pigs, lambs, and cows have higher levels of omega-3 fatty acid (an anti-inflammatory fat) and lower levels of omega-6 fatty acid (a pro-inflammatory fat). Not unexpectedly, evidence has linked consuming meat from grass-fed animals to a lower risk of disease than meat from corn-fed animals. There are other health advantages of purchasing certified organic meats, or meat that is certified to be free of growth hormones and antibiotics, if feasible. Hormone and antibiotic compounds fed to livestock end up in our foods, upsetting our endocrine system, potentially inducing hormone-dependent cancers (such as breast, cervical, and prostate cancer), and contributing to the global proliferation of antibiotic-resistant microbes like methicillin-resistant Staphylococcus aureus (MRSA).

Since too much pork isn't grass-fed, free-range, or sustainable, the next option will be to cut down on your intake.

Brassicas, cruciferous vegetables, and leafy greens

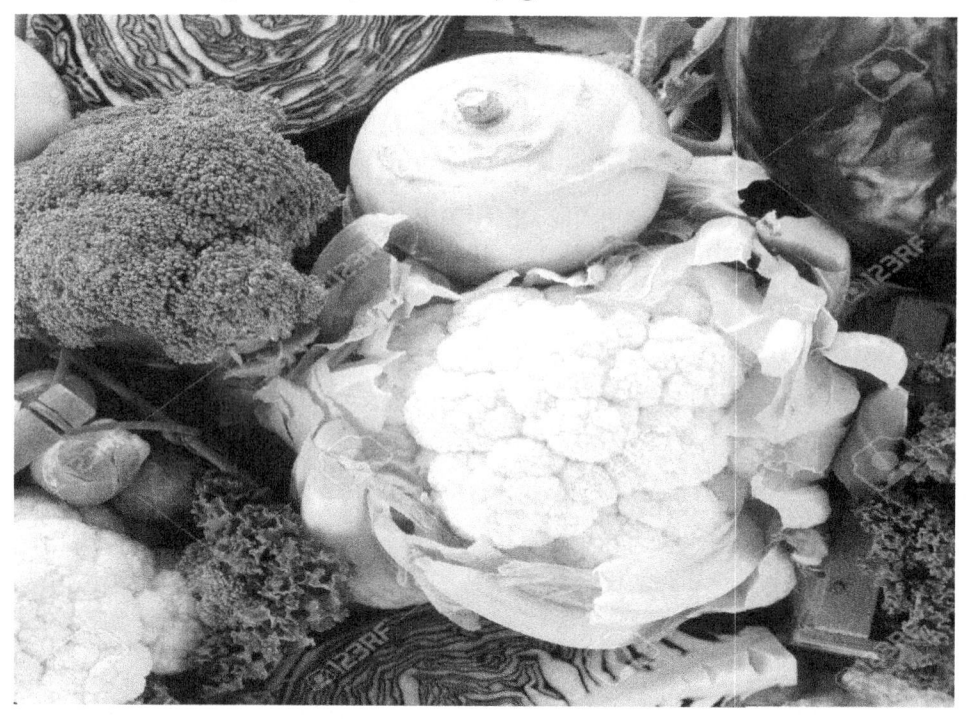

Arugula, collard greens, bok choy, daikon radish, broccoli, Chinese cabbage, Brussels sprouts, cabbage, cauliflower, kale, horseradish, turnip, kohlrabi, rutabaga, mustard greens, and watercress are all examples of cruciferous vegetables. These vegetables are classified as superfoods because they are rich in antioxidants, including vitamin C and manganese. They're both a good source of fiber and protein. Sulforaphane, contained in these vegetables, helps to reduce inflammation by speeding up step two detoxification in the liver. Broccoli, for example, has two-thirds the protein of a chicken breast and 9 grams of fiber. If you're searching for the ideal cancer-fighting meal, look no further than cruciferous vegetables. Multiple experiments have discovered that glucosinolates, a form of compound contained in these vegetables, have potent anti-cancer properties.

Kale, in addition to other cruciferous vegetables and leafy greens, merits a special mention due to its recent success.

Chefs love kale because it's simple to produce and cook with. Kale stems, ranging from chips to premade salads, can be found on the shelves of several supermarkets. With the spotlight, you might be shocked to hear that kale produces a lot of oxalic acids, which can induce kidney stones and interfere with calcium absorption as it builds up in the body. (Fun fact: the plant does this to defend itself from predators.) Instead of consuming kale fresh, lightly steam it for around 5 minutes to inactivate the oxalic acid and improve the vast nutritional advantages, including cholesterol-lowering properties. Split the leaves and stems into 1/4- to 1/2-in [6- to 12-mm] slices to ensure even cooking and better chewing.

Kale's cancer-prevention properties come from its high concentration of carotenoids and flavonoids, which are potent antioxidants, as well as isothiocyanates, which have been shown to enhance both phase 1 and phase 2 of the liver's detoxification pathway, resulting in a massive increase in the body's detoxification ability.

Dark chocolate

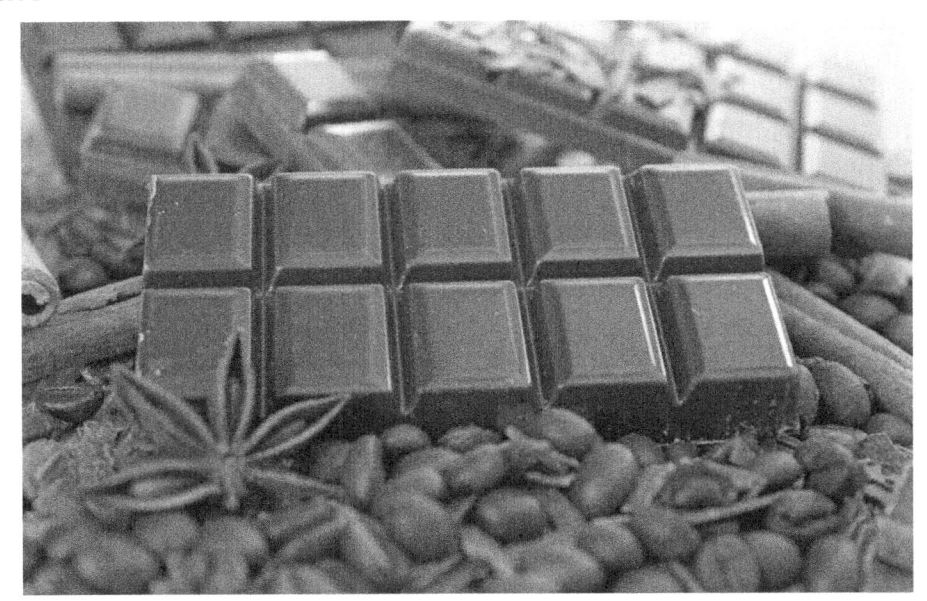

Doctors prescribe dark chocolate (70 percent cocoa or more) as the first guilt-free snack. It has been shown to be beneficial to the pancreas, heart, and gastrointestinal system in studies (ground zero for inflammation). If eaten consistently in limited amounts, it increases the body's reaction to a glucose sugar–enriched meal by improving insulin sensitivity, eventually slowing or avoiding the development of prediabetes and diabetes. The fibrous cacao particles that aren't digested help your intestinal bacteria thrive. According to studies, 1 oz [30 g] of dark chocolate with a cacao content of 70% or higher increases coronary function in healthier persons and cardiovascular patients by increasing arterial blood supply and reducing blood pressure modestly.

Turmeric & Other Dried Spices

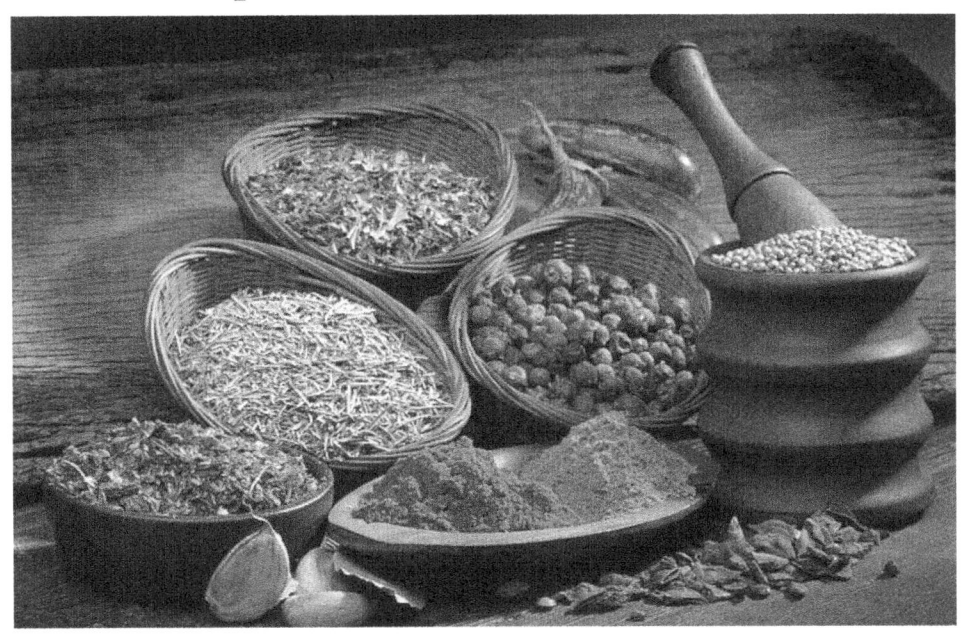

Spices have also been used to enhance the flavor of food while still providing nutritional benefits. Confucius advocated for the use of young, roasted, and ground ginger with any meal for digestive benefits. Spice is more often thought of as a flavoring agent, but it often benefits the body, brings texture to sauces, and replaces heavy salt or sugar use.

Cinnamon has been shown to minimize bloating and discomfort-causing bacteria in the digestive tract, improve general circulation and control blood sugar levels during meals. Turmeric has been shown to be an effective anti-inflammatory and anti-cancer agent, making it an excellent addition to foods for those who have arthritis or cancer. Turmeric is available in capsule form at health food stores, but my preferred method of consuming it is by sprinkling it on savory dishes. Black pepper, like many other spices, serves as a thermogenic, boosting the metabolic rate and double the absorption of turmeric and other compounds with low bioavailability (natural tendency to be consumed by the body).

Fish: salmon and other oily types

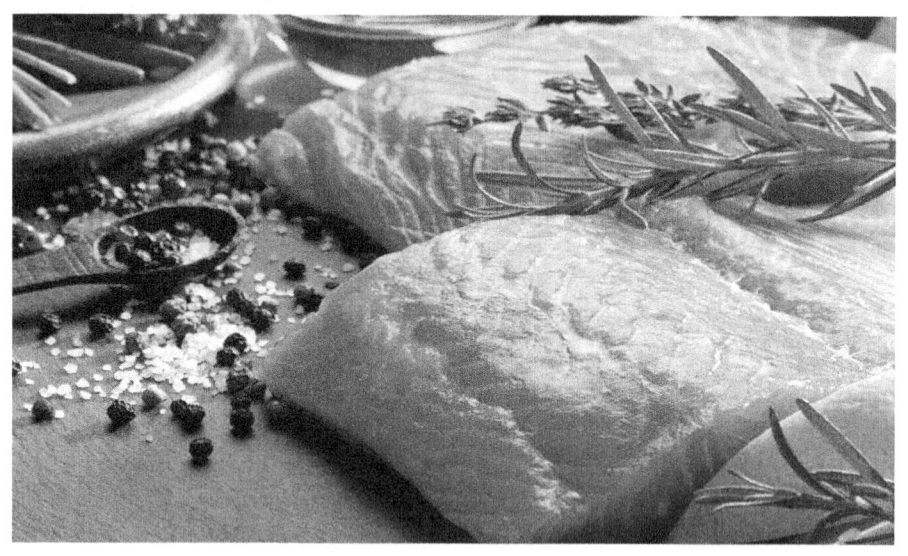

Adults and children can consume three servings of cold-water fish each week, particularly pregnant women. Cold-water fish including salmon, black cod (sable fish), rainbow trout, anchovies, whitefish, Atlantic mackerel, Atlantic herring, and Pacific sardines have low mercury levels and polyunsaturated solid fatty acid content. Omega-3 fatty acids have been shown to decrease inflammation, enhance cardiac wellbeing, inflammatory diseases, and mood disorders, and encourage skin and nail health. They're genuinely a miracle meal. Countless people have seen significant improvements in their pain-related symptoms after consuming a consistent diet of cold-water seafood. Stop feeding top-of-the-food-chain fish such as sharks, swordfish, tilefish, and king mackerel to reduce mercury toxicity.

Green Tea

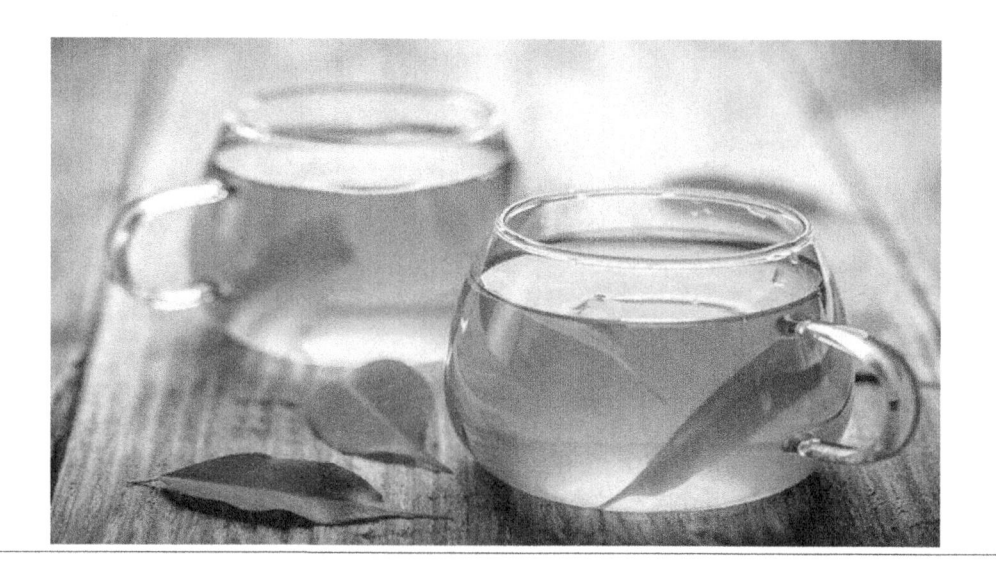

Green tea leaves are not fermented, but they have more polyphenols than oolong or black tea leaves.

Polyphenols are essential antioxidants, with epigallocatechin gallate being the most well-known. Green tea often includes alkaloids including caffeine, theophylline (used to treat asthma), and theobromine (used in toothpaste for its antimicrobial properties), both of which contribute to the tea's energizing impact. The amino acid L-theanine, found in tea, has been shown to increase mental clarity and calm nerves. Green tea's medicinal advantages are well established in conventional healing practices; it promotes heart health, extracts extra fat from the body, balances blood pressure, improves metabolism, and calms the mind when used as a daily remedy. According to recent research, consuming three cups of tea a day reduces the incidence of cancer, cardiac attack, and stroke by 20 to 30%. As if that weren't enough, research shows that green tea will boost metabolism and encourage the body to kill fat cells first, resulting in weight loss.

Legumes

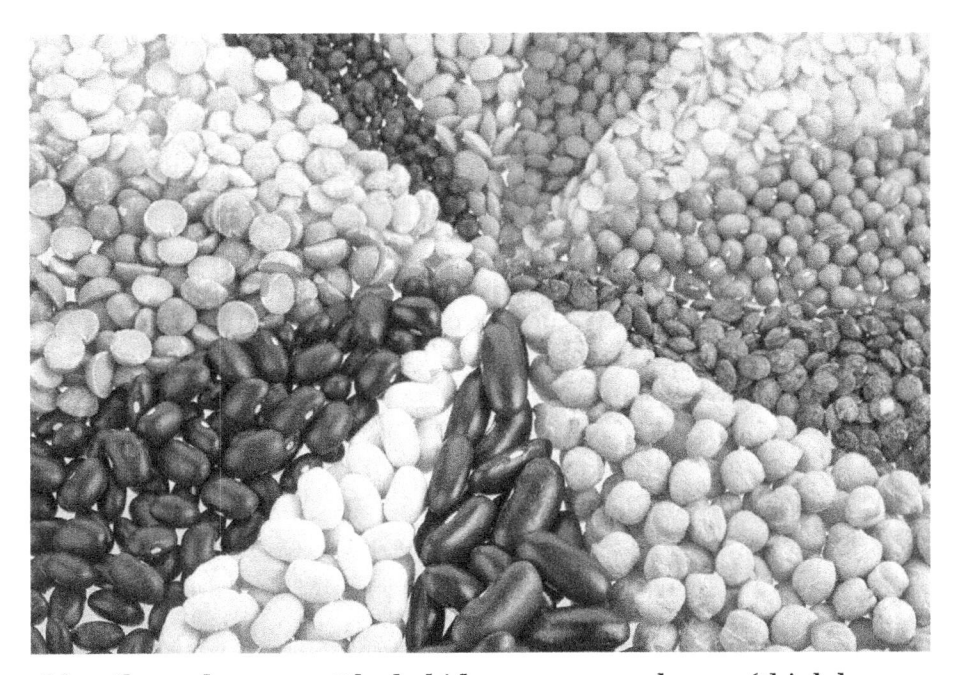

Peas, beans, and lentils are legumes. Black, kidney, navy, garbanzo (think hummus), and soy are only a few of the options (think tofu and tempeh). Both are high in fiber, iron, protein, zinc, calcium, and B vitamins, and phytochemicals tend to reduce inflammation. Cooked black beans (1 cup [170 g]) have 15 grams of fiber and protein (more than the average American gets in an entire day). Cooked lentils have 30 grams of fiber and 25 grams of protein in 1/2 cup [125 g], making them an ideal alternative for vegetarians or others trying to reduce their meat intake.

Garbanzo beans are a good option for those who want to improve their folate and manganese intake. Cooked garbanzos have 14 grams of fiber and protein per cup [250 g].

While much controversy in the media regarding the dangers and advantages of soy, research proves that it is a superior food supply. Soymilk, soybeans (edamame), tempeh, tofu, miso, soy "meat," and soy "cheese" are only a few examples. These types of soy protein are superior to the more refined and manufactured soy protein used in energy bars and powders. Soy is high in carbohydrates, polyunsaturated fat, vitamins, protein, and minerals while being deficient in saturated fat.

Natural Sweetener

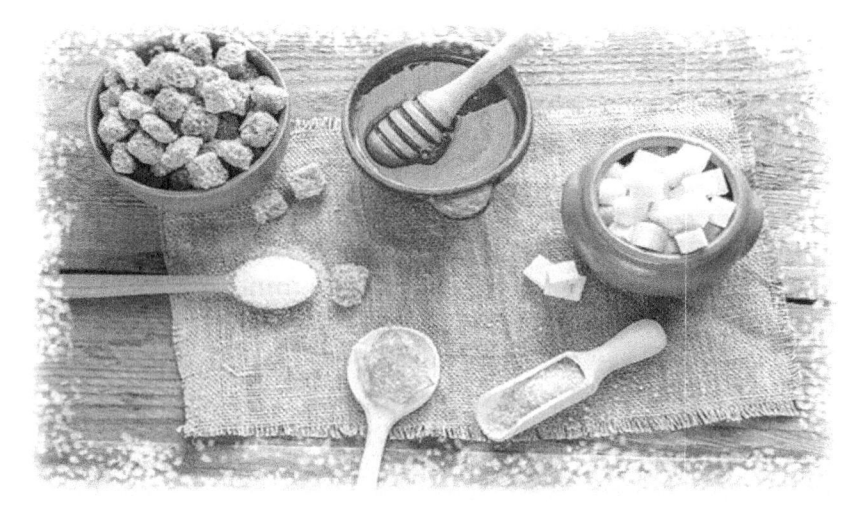

Natural sweeteners also share one thing in common: they're essentially sugars that you introduce to your food, and as such, they can be used in moderation. The distinctions between sweeteners like cane sugar, agave, maple syrup, and white sugar, with the exception of honey, are minor. As a result, choose flavor over food content, opt for herbal versions to avoid contaminants in addition to sugar, and use the smallest volume of sugar available to sweeten treats.

Agave syrup is made from blue agave fruit, which is often used to make tequila. It has a sweeter flavor than beet or cane sugar but a lower glycaemic index (the measure of how a carbohydrate-containing food increases glucose in the blood). Isn't this too amazing to be true? Unfortunately, this is the case. Since agave produces heavily refined fructose (think high-fructose corn syrup), which is difficult for the liver to digest and may contribute to fatty liver and obesity, it has less sugar but tastes sweeter. Fructose use is a significant contributor to the Western world's growing fatty liver crisis. In comparison to white sugar, agave has 60 calories per 1 tablespoon.

Honey seems to provide the most health advantages of the natural sweeteners, promising to cure skin wounds, reduce cough and diarrhea in children (give only to children age two and older), and mitigate the symptoms of environmental allergies, to mention a handful.

Maple syrup contains more than 54 antioxidants (more than double as much as processed sugars), although you'd have to eat a lot of it to enjoy any of the benefits. In comparison to the harm done to your body from all those additional carbohydrates, the nutritional input will be marginal. Honey and maple syrup are the sweeteners of choice when it comes to applying sweetness to the fruit.

Quinoa

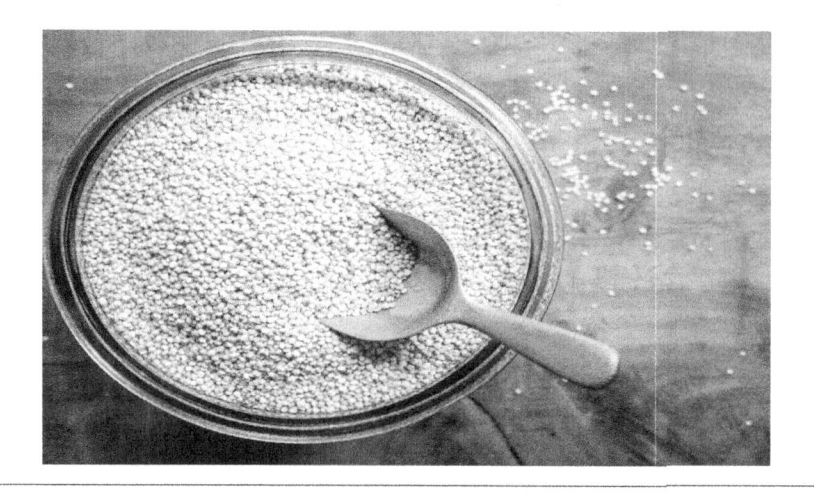

Quinoa, a gluten-free meal that can be eaten as a grain but is still the seed of the plant, has been a staple in South America for over 5,000 years. Since it has an excellent protein-to-carbohydrate ratio, is a total protein (meaning it doesn't need to be combined with another compound to supply protein to the body), is high in healthy fats and fiber, and is a complex carbohydrate, it was deemed an ideal food for astronauts. As a consequence, it contains all of the macro and micronutrients that you need in a meal. It has anti-inflammatory and antioxidant properties, increases blood sugar control, reduces LDL cholesterol, and functions as a short- and long-term fuel source. Rinse quinoa thoroughly before cooking to extract saponins, a naturally occurring pesticide that gives the grain a bitter flavor.

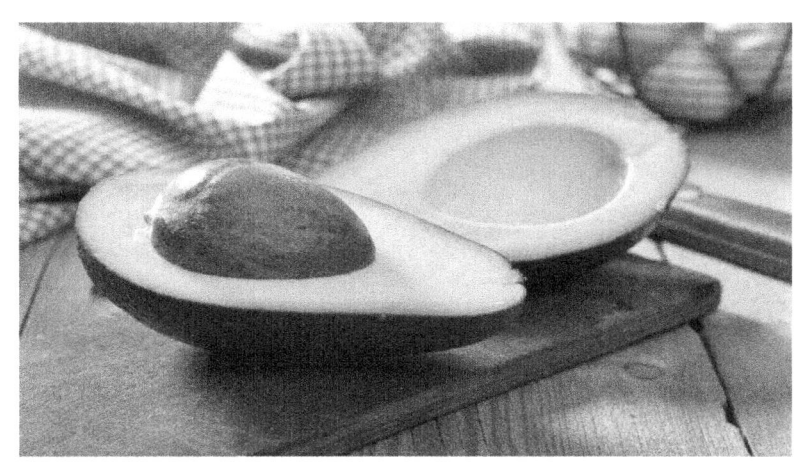

Avocados

Avocados are high in mono- and polyunsaturated fats, phytosterols, alpha-linolenic acid (omega-3 fatty acids), and carotenoids, which have many health benefits. Avocados have been shown to decrease inflammation, blood sugar elevation, and cholesterol, as well as the symptoms of osteoarthritis and rheumatoid arthritis, according to research. Avocado's moisturizing oils and fats often help to tone skin and moisturize hair. Avocado is an excellent substitute for other oils and fats in cooking; use it where butter or mayonnaise will generally be used. Avocado contains 227 calories, 9 grams of fiber, 3 grams of protein, and 21 grams of fat, 75 percent of which are healthy mono- and polyunsaturated fats. Alpha- and beta-carotene, zeaxanthin, lutein, neochrome, neoxanthin, and chrysanthemaxanthin are some of the carotenoids contained in avocado. Many of these substances often help to delay the onset of vision disorders, including macular degeneration. Avocado's high-fat content means that adding avocado to a salad increases the absorption of antioxidant carotenoids in the salad by 200 to 400 percent.

Citrus fruits

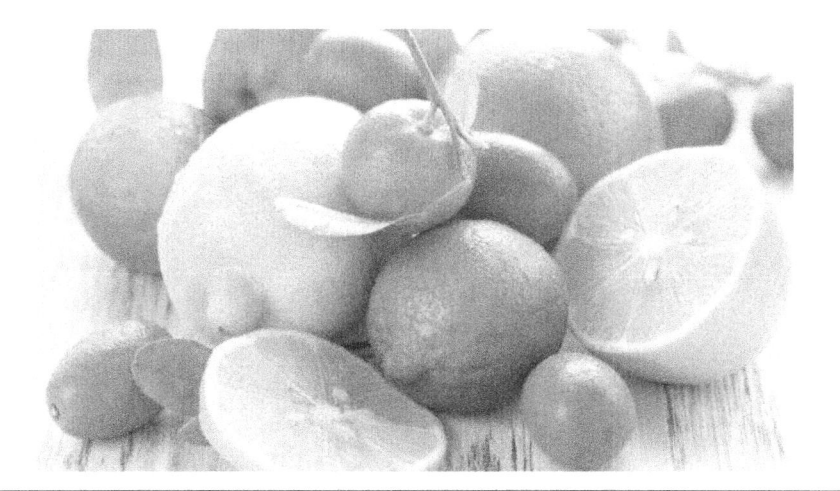

Citrus fruits, especially grapefruits, limes, clementine, lemons, and oranges, are health warriors in any form. During the cold season, we usually applaud citrus for its strong vitamin C content, but there's so much more to love about it.

Every form of citrus can offer hydration and electrolytes to thirsty bodies due to their high-water content. Citrus flavonoids have also been shown to neutralize free radicals, perhaps inhibiting cancer cell proliferation. The skin, as well as the juice and flesh, contain anti-inflammatory effects.

Dried chiles

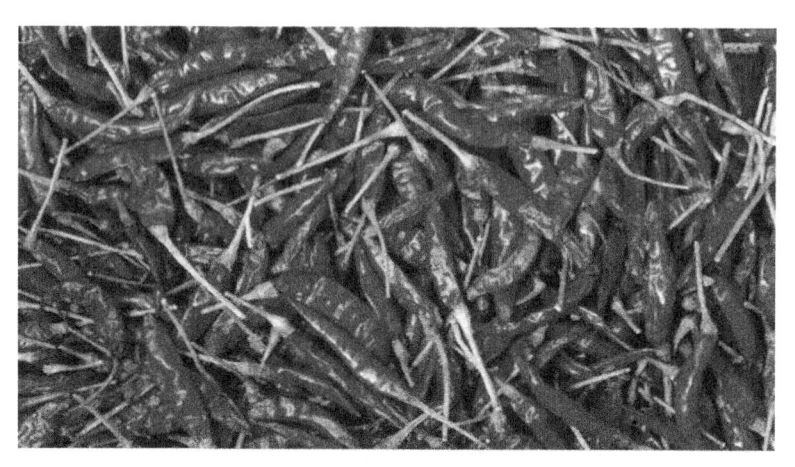

Nightshades, which have chiles, may be dangerous for those who suffer from inflammatory disorders. If nightshades or, more accurately, chiles do not bother you, then chiles can be helpful to you. The capsaicin content of dried chiles such as chipotle, ancho, and guajillo is what gives them their heat. Capsaicin is a well-known potent pain reliever and anti-inflammatory agent that, when taken daily, lowers the risk of developing diabetes.

Capsaicin inhibits the neuropeptide substance P, which can help to relieve nerve and joint discomfort. Companies market capsaicin lotions and patches for the management of joint discomforts, such as osteoarthritis and neuropathic pain caused by diabetes and sciatica, based on the study. (Because capsaicin is painful to apply at first, people can feel discomfort before experiencing relief.) Furthermore, studies have shown that people who eat dried chiles raise their metabolic rate for 30 minutes, needless insulin in response to a carbohydrate-rich meal, and avoid triglyceride and cholesterol oxidation (free radical production). Capsaicin is concentrated in the flesh and seeds of the pepper, so use the seeds only if you can tolerate the sun. The higher the capsaicin level, the hotter the pepper.

Eggs

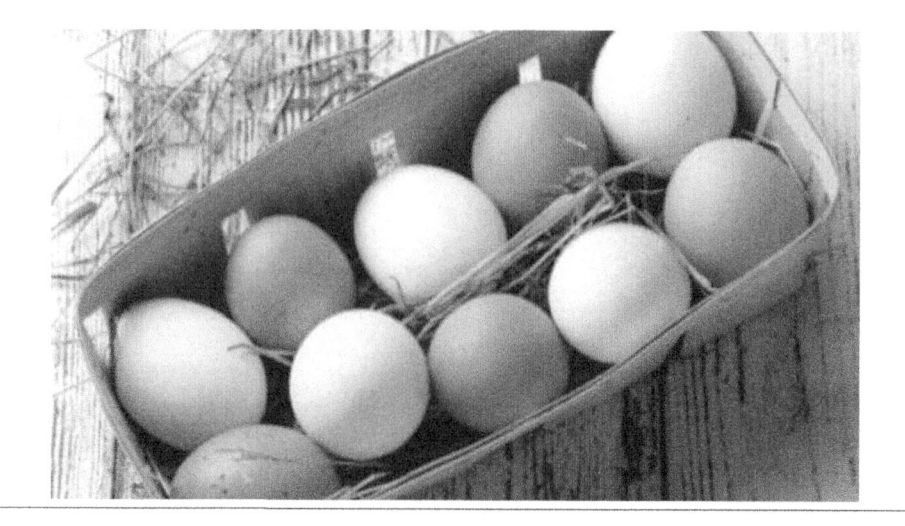

Because of their high protein, vitamin A and B, and biotin quality, many doctors refer to eggs as the "perfect meal." Since eggs include the powerful carotenoids zeaxanthin and lutein (both good for vision), as well as choline, they tend to reduce inflammation (good for brain and heart function). The first law of eating these oval powerhouses is to purchase organic wherever possible. Organic eggs are richer in omega-3 fatty acids and are free of antibiotic compounds such as Tylenol, Benadryl, and arsenic, which are introduced to the feed of conventionally raised poultry and can be found in low amounts in the product. (Arsenic, yes!) It's commonly added to the feed mix by conventional farmers to avoid infections.) The second maxim is to avoid being duped by deceptive marketing tactics; "pasture-raised" and "cage-free" are not synonymous! Though buying from local farmers who take pride in raising free-roaming hens is still the best choice, pasture-raised is a close second. Simply placed, real pasture-raised hens are raised in open fields and encouraged to forage for their own food. Cage-free or sometimes "free-range" hens are often shifted from cage to cage or granted brief periods outside. The usage of such health-halo logos is only permitted due to regulatory loopholes.

Garlic and Onions

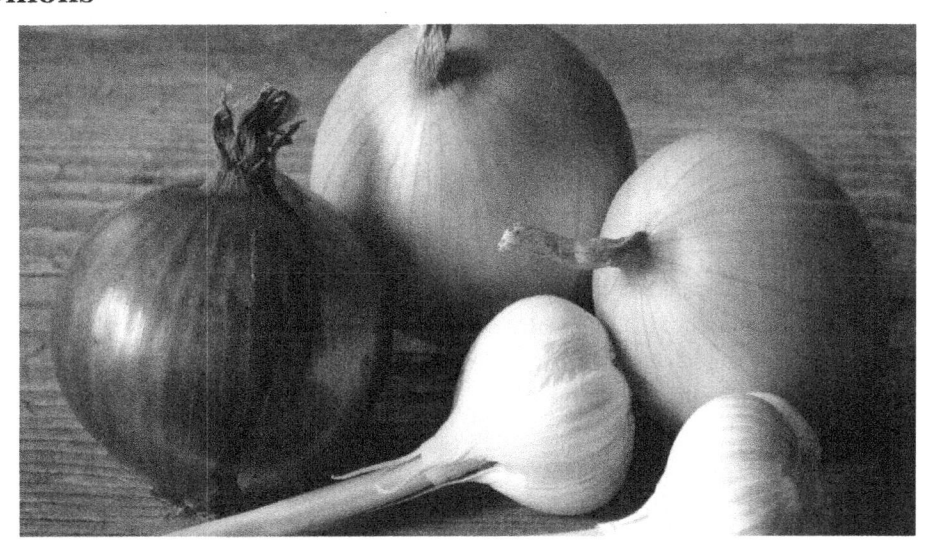

These and other short-chain fructooligosaccharides (scFOS) are sweet, low-calorie carbohydrates that are tasty.

Since these things aren't fully digested in the stomach, the leftover content feeds the good bacteria that live there, resulting in a cleaner gut. These foods often improve the immune system and reduce inflammation as a result of this mechanism. The flavor of scFOS is about twice that of table sugar, albeit without the calories. Other foods that include scFOS include asparagus, leeks, jicama roots, Jerusalem artichokes, burdock roots, chicory, and dandelion roots, in addition to onions and garlic. Garlic, also known as the stinking rose, belongs to the allium genus, which also contains leeks and onions. Sulphur compounds (allicin, alliin, 1, 2-vinyldithin, hydrogen sulphide) are responsible for many of the health effects, including decreased inflammation and oxidation, as well as modestly decreasing oxidized cholesterols, triglycerides, blood pressure, and blood clotting. Garlic can also shield you from cancer. Manganese, selenium, and vitamin B6 are all contained in it.

Purchase garlic fresh (rather than flakes or powder), cut it and set it aside for 10 to 15 minutes to enable the alliinase enzymes to work before using it in a recipe for maximum health benefits. While garlic is best eaten fresh, many people have trouble tolerating it; if this is the case with you, add the garlic near the end of the cooking phase to reduce its digestive effect.

Herbs

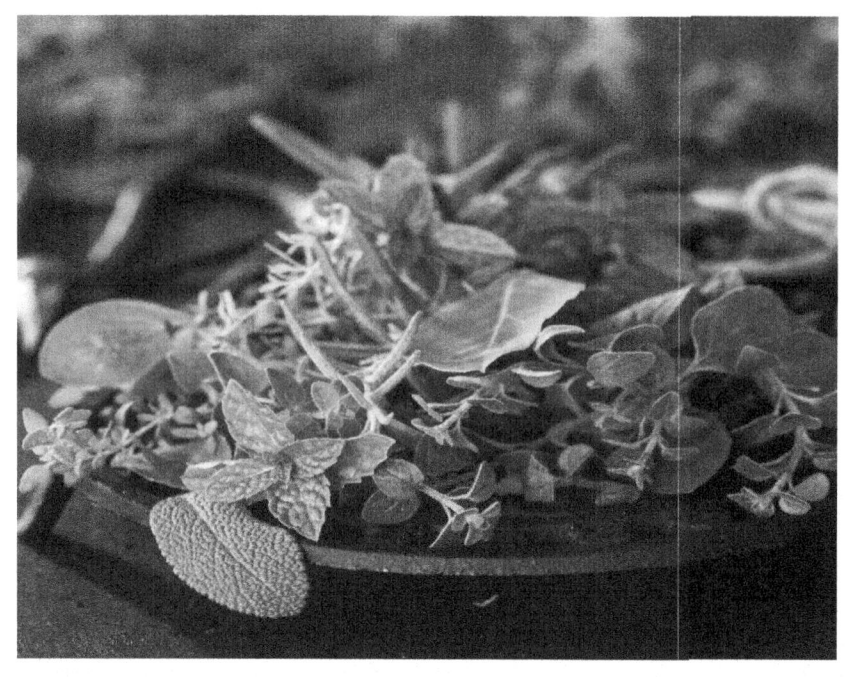

Herbs have been valued since antiquity because they not only give spice to a multitude of dishes, but they are often superfoods. Oregano, as a leafy weed, has a lot of antioxidant properties. Oregano oil is a natural antibiotic that has been used for centuries. The addition of rosemary or lavender to a dish will help to ease anxiety, discomfort and boost mood. Parsley is more than just a garnish; in laboratory experiments, the volatile oils have been shown to inhibit the development of cancer cells. Moroccans set a strong example for the rest of us by drinking tea made from a mint infusion to help digestion and cleanse the palate, which has anti-inflammatory effects.

Mushrooms

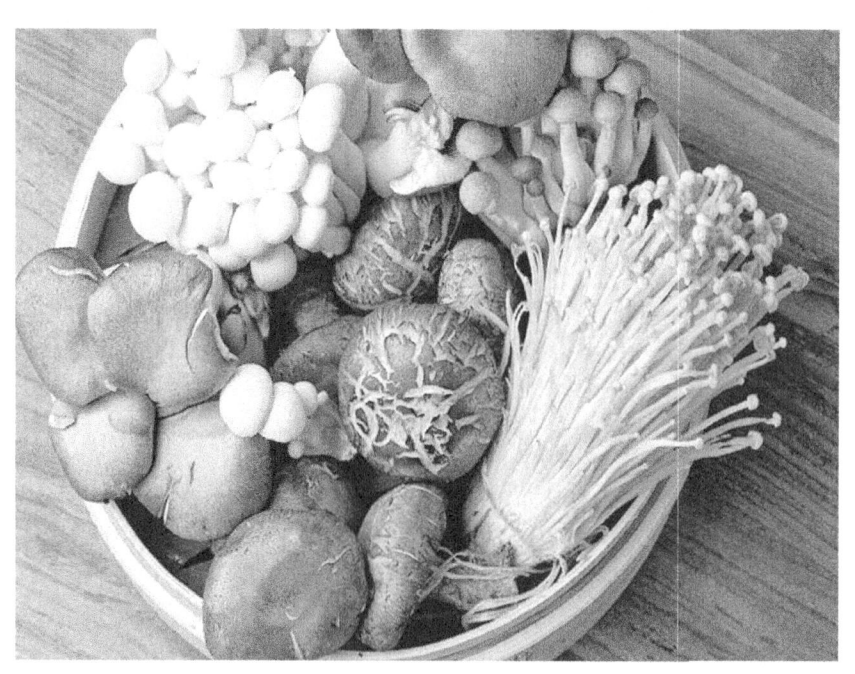

Mushrooms have incredible health-promoting properties. These wonder foods are available in a bewildering variety of edible forms.

Since they thrive in wet soil, they ingest both good and bad elements, so organic is better. Mushrooms are a hearty and heart-healthy meat alternative that often carries vitamins and minerals. Mushroom supplements are available for a variety of health benefits, but consuming them is the safest way to begin. Cremini, shiitake, reishi "spirit plant," turkey tail, "cloud," and white button are among my favorites. They're all suitable for the immune system and have anti-inflammatory properties.

Oils

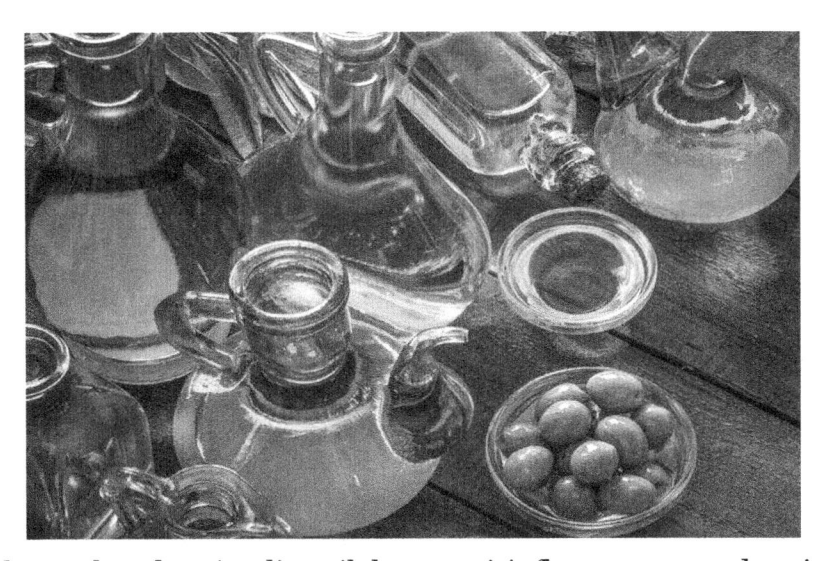

Polyphenols, which are abundant in olive oil, have anti-inflammatory and antioxidant properties. Any of the preparation can be done with extra-virgin olive oil (from the first pressing). More than 70% of its fat comes from oleic acid, a monounsaturated fat that has been shown to lower blood pressure, lower LDL (bad) cholesterol, and raise HDL (good) cholesterol, among other heart-healthy properties. Canola oil comes near, with monounsaturated fat accounting for 60% of the fat content.

When coconut oil was heavily refined and had partly hydrogenated oil, among other unhealthful chemicals, it gained a poor name in the 1980s. Fresh-pressed coconut oil, which is now available in raw form (rather than in refined foods), is a healthy option (albeit less so than olive oil or canola oil). While coconut oil contains 90% saturated fat (compared to 64% in butter), virgin and processed coconut oil, unlike butter, contains saturated fat in the form of lauric acid, a medium-chain triglyceride. Lauric acid has been found to improve HDL cholesterol levels and be a readily digestible source of continuous energy for the elderly and athletes.

Seeds

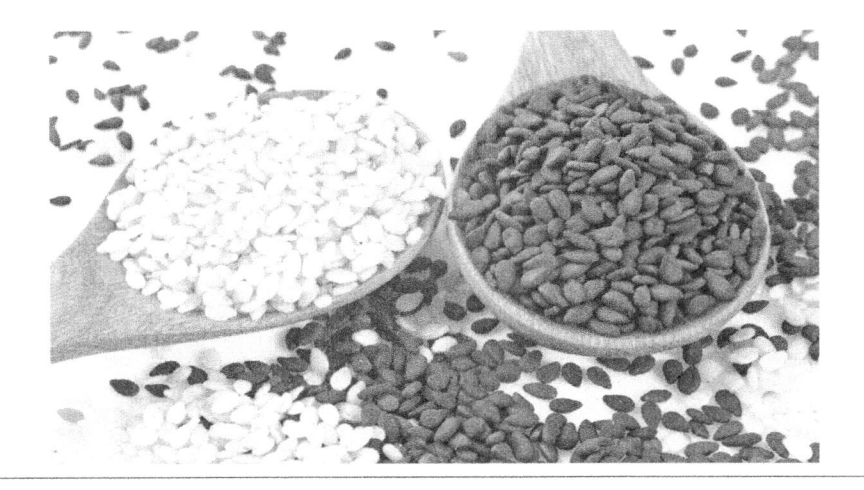

Seeds like sesame, sunflower, pumpkin, and others are high in healthy fats, fiber, and protein. Manganese, magnesium (helps with PMS and blood pressure), vitamin B6 (supports nerve function and heart health), potassium (lowers blood pressure), the whole spectrum of vitamin E (supports heart health and reduces cancer risk), zinc (promotes the immune system and prostate health), plant-based omega-3 fatty acids (treats autoimmune conditions), plant sterols (lowers cholesterol and promotes prostate health), and other vital nutrients. According to studies, consuming a tiny handful of seeds every day of the week will help lower blood sugar levels, increase cholesterol, reduce the risk of heart disease, improve metabolism, and lower cancer risk.

Tree Nuts

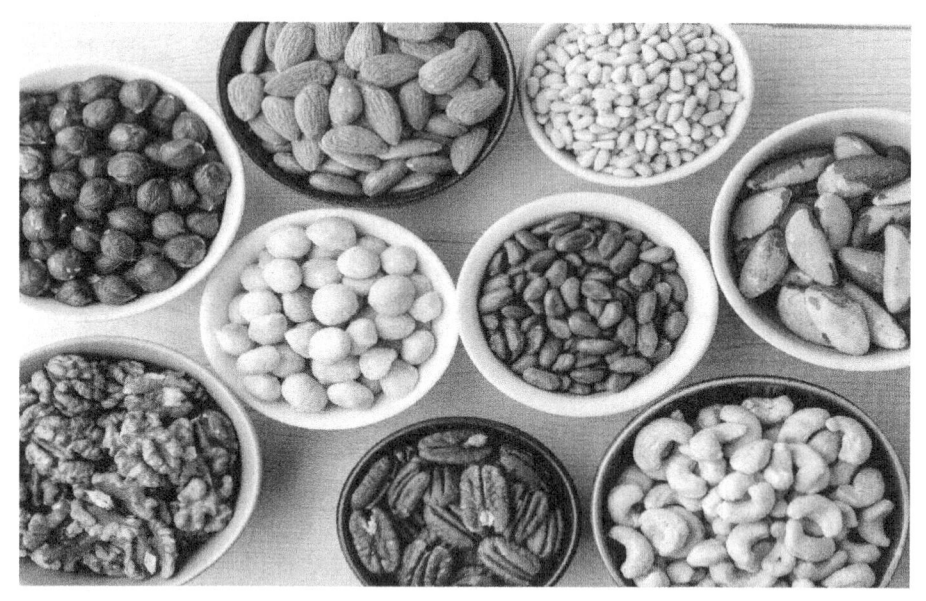

Almonds, chestnuts, cashews, hazelnuts, pistachios, pecans, and walnuts, whether raw or toasted, are high in healthy fats, fiber, protein, and antioxidants. Nuts, when eaten many days a week as a snack, have long-lasting nutrition. A Mediterranean diet that includes a small handful of nuts or one tablespoon of nut butter four times a week has been shown to lower blood sugar levels following a carbohydrate-heavy meal, lower LDL cholesterol, and decrease the risk of heart disease by 30%.

Nuts can have a sustained energy boost, thus leaving you feeling complete and happy. The maximum antioxidant content of all tree nuts is found in chestnuts, pecans, and walnuts (which are rich in omega-3 fatty acids).

Sweet Potatoes

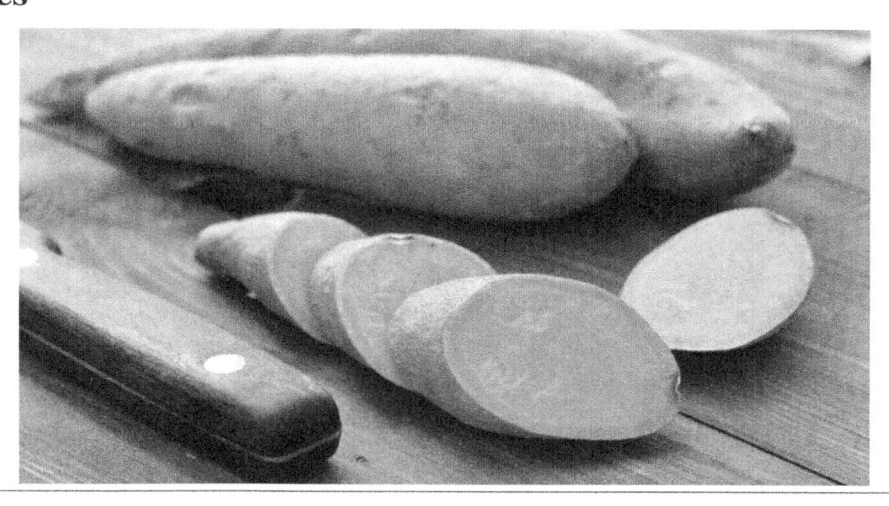

Sweet potatoes, with many of their variations, are much more nutritious than their pale equivalent, the white potato. Our taste buds are not deceitful. There's a reason caramelized sweet potatoes taste so good: they're practically candy! To get the most nutritional benefits from sweet potatoes while still controlling their sugar content, cook them only long enough to soften but not mushy. When a sweet potato caramelizes (and becomes mushy), the fiber breaks down, allowing the potato to be quickly digested in the same manner as an essential starch is.

Like white bread and pasta, russet potatoes are an essential starch or carbohydrate that can be eaten in moderation. They break down quickly into sugar when eaten, while sweet potatoes, which are a complicated starch or carbohydrate, require longer to digest. As a consequence, the sugar takes longer to reach the bloodstream, resulting in a slower spike in blood sugar and a more gradual rise in insulin levels. Easy starches are much more likely than complex starches to cause insulin resistance and diabetes over time. To get the most vitamins and minerals, eat the skins of every kind of potato whenever possible.

Anti-inflammatory Foods				
Vegetables	**Fruits/Nuts/Seeds**	**Meats/Fish/Eggs**	**Herbs/Spices/Tea**	**Healthy Fats**
kale spinach Swiss chard collard greens bok choy celery beets broccoli peppers avocados onions fermented vegetables shiitake mushrooms tomatoes black beans raw oats brown rice amaranth millet	blueberries strawberries cherries oranges apples pineapple watermelon almonds walnuts chia seeds flax seeds	*fatty fish:* *salmon *mackerel *tuna *sardines other wild-caught fish oysters grass-fed meats pastured organic eggs bone broth	green tea matcha tea tulsi tea garlic ginger cayenne rosemary turmeric cinnamon oregano clove nutmeg sage thyme coffee	olive oil coconut oil MCT oil ghee grass-fed butter

Chapter 5- Food Shopping List for Anti-Inflammatory Diet

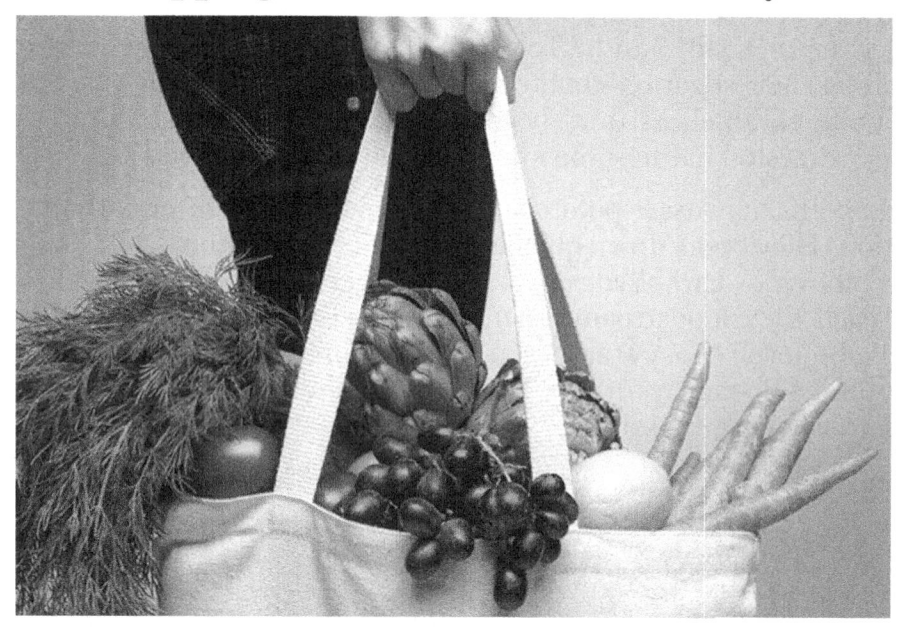

5.1 The Anti-Inflammatory Shopping List

Whenever you go grocery shopping, you should keep in mind the recipes that you are going to make in the week. The grocery shopping can either be done weekly or daily depending upon the distance of the grocery store from your place or the availability of fresh produce. The quantity of the products can change according to the portions you are making.

1st and 2nd Week Shopping list

Fresh Produce

- Arugula, five cups
- Avocados, 3
- Beets, 2
- Celeriac (celery root), one medium
- Chard, three bunches
- Garlic, two heads
- Grapes, one bunch
- Kale, four bunches
- Limes, 2
- Pear, 1
- Portobello mushrooms, 3
- Shallots, three small
- Spinach, six cups
- Apples, 2

- Asparagus, 1 pound
- Banana, 1
- Carrots, 6
- Celery, one head
- Cremini mushrooms, half-pound
- Garnet yams, 3
- Ginger, 1 (1-inch) piece
- Green onions, two bunches
- Lemons, 3
- Mango, 1
- Pomegranate, 1
- Red onion, 1
- Shiitake mushrooms, 1 pound
- Strawberries, 3
- Yellow onions, 3
- Sunchokes (Jerusalem artichokes), 4

Frozen Foods
- Mango, one cup chopped
- Peas, 3/4 cup
- Mixed berries, one cup

Fish, Meat, and Poultry
- Lamb sausages, 2
- Salmon, one and a half pounds
- Whitefish (black cod, cod, or halibut), one and a half pounds
- Anchovies, 4, or anchovy paste, 1 to 2 teaspoons
- Light fish (cod, halibut, or red snapper), one and a half pounds
- Sardines, 1 pound fresh

Cereals, Grains, and Flours
- Oats, one and a half cups certified gluten-free
- Rainbow quinoa, 1 cup
- Brown rice flour, 3/4 cup
- Quinoa flour, two cups

Nuts, Seeds, and Dried Fruits

- Almonds, 1 cup raw
- Brazil nuts, half cup
- Cherries, half cup dried
- Dates, half cup pitted
- Mangoes, half cup dried (unsweetened and unsulfured)
- Pistachios, one and a half cups shelled
- Almond butter, half cup
- Blueberries, half cup freeze-dried
- Cashews, 3/4 cup raw
- Chia seeds, a quarter cup
- Hazelnuts, 3/4 cup
- Pine nuts, a quarter cup
- Pumpkin seeds (pepitas), one and a half cups shelled
- Walnuts, two cups
- Tahini (sesame seed paste), one tablespoon

Herbs and Spices

- Bay leaf, 1
- Cardamom, half teaspoon ground
- Celery seed, one teaspoon
- Cinnamon, two tablespoons ground
- Curry powder, two teaspoons
- Mint, four leaves
- Oregano, one tablespoon fresh, or two teaspoons dried
- Sage, one teaspoon dried
- Basil, 4 to 5 large leaves or two teaspoons dried
- Black peppercorns
- Cayenne pepper, 1/8 teaspoon
- Cilantro, one bunch
- Cumin, one tablespoon ground
- Fenugreek, half teaspoon dried
- Nutmeg, half teaspoon ground
- Parsley, one bunch

- Sea salt
- Turmeric, one teaspoon ground
- Thyme, one tablespoon fresh, or two teaspoons dried

Oils and Vinegar
- Champagne vinegar, one tablespoon
- Extra-virgin olive oil, 1 (16-ounce) bottle
- Sunflower oil (optional), one tablespoon
- Balsamic vinegar, two tablespoons
- Coconut oil, a quarter cup
- Grapeseed oil, 1 (12-ounce) bottle

Sweeteners
- Agave nectar, three teaspoons
- Maple syrup, two tablespoons
- Honey, two teaspoons

Other
- Almond extract, 1/8 teaspoon
- Baby lima beans, one cup dried
- Baking soda, half teaspoon
- Cannellini or other white beans, one (15-ounce) can
- Chickpeas (garbanzo beans), one (15-ounce) can
- Coconut milk, 1 cup unsweetened
- French lentils, half cup dried
- Green olives, one and a half cups
- Kalamata olives, 3 cups pitted
- Adzuki beans, 1 (15-ounce) can
- Almond milk, 1 cup unsweetened Artichoke heart marinated in olive oil, 1 (14-ounce) jar
- Baking powder, two tablespoons
- Black beans, 1 (15-ounce) can
- Capers, two teaspoons
- Coconut, half cup unsweetened and shredded
- Cooking sherry, two tablespoons
- Golden raisins, a quarter cup
- Hemp milk (optional), half cup unsweetened

- Kombu (optional), 1 (2-ounce) package
- Vegetable broth, six cups
- Mushroom broth, 1 quart

3rd Week Shopping list

Fresh Produce

- Avocados, 2
- Banana, 1
- Broccoli, two heads
- Celery, one head
- Cremini mushrooms, 1 pound
- Garlic, one head
- Jicama, one small
- Kale, two bunches
- Pears, 2
- Red onion, one small
- Apples, 2
- Baby spinach or baby kale, two cups
- Beets, 2
- Carrots, 14
- Chard, one bunch
- Fresh spinach, ½ pound
- Ginger, 1 (1-inch piece)
- Kaffir lime leaves, 5 (or buy two limes for zest and juice if lime leaves are not available)
- Lemon, 1
- Radishes, 10
- Scallions or green onions, one bunch
- Yellow onions, two small
- Spaghetti squash, one small

Frozen Foods

- Mixed berries, 1 (10-ounce) bag
- Mangoes, 1 (10-ounce) bag
- Petite peas, 3 (10-ounce) bags

Fish, Meat, and Poultry
- Whitefish (black cod, cod, or halibut), 1 pound
- Halibut, one and a half pounds

Cereals, Grains, and Flours
- Brown rice flour, a quarter cup
- Quinoa, 1 cup
- Brown rice, a quarter cup
- Oats, 5half cups certified gluten-free

Nuts, Seeds, and Dried Fruits
- Brazil nuts, half cup
- Chia seeds, half cup
- Hazelnuts, 1 cup
- Pine nuts, a quarter cup
- Sesame seeds, 1⁄4 raw
- Walnuts, one and a half cups
- Almond butter, half cup
- Cashews, quarter cup raw
- Currants, half cup dried
- Pecans, 3⁄4 cup
- Pumpkin seeds (pepitas), 1 cup shelled
- Sunflower seeds, 3⁄4 cup

Herbs and Spices
- Black peppercorns
- Cayenne pepper, a quarter teaspoon
- Cumin, three teaspoons ground
- Dill, one teaspoon dried
- Italian herbs, half cup dried
- Nutmeg, half teaspoon ground
- Basil, 4 to 5 leaves, and one teaspoon dried
- Cardamom, half teaspoon ground
- Cinnamon, one teaspoon ground
- Curry powder, two teaspoons
- Fenugreek, half teaspoon dried

- Mint, four leaves
- Oregano, one teaspoon dried
- Turmeric, one teaspoon ground
- Sea salt

Oils and Vinegar
- Balsamic vinegar, two tablespoons
- Apple cider vinegar, one tablespoon
- Coconut oil, 3/4 cup
- Grapeseed oil, three tablespoons
- Extra-virgin olive oil, 1 (16-ounce) bottle

Sweeteners
- Coconut palm sugar, half cup
- Agave nectar, a quarter cup
- Honey, one and a half teaspoons

Other
- Black beans, half cup
- Chickpeas (garbanzo beans), 1 (15-ounce) can
- Dijon or stone-ground mustard, half teaspoon
- Green olives, half cup
- Kalamata olives, half cup pitted
- Artichoke hearts marinated in olive oil, 1 (14-ounce) jar
- Cannellini beans, 1 (15-ounce) can
- Coconut milk, two cups
- Dill pickles, 1 (8-ounce) jar
- Hemp or almond milk, half cup unsweetened
- Pumpkin puree, 1 (15-ounce) can
- Vegetable broth, 4 quarts
- Vegenaise, 1 cup soy-free

4th Week Shopping List

Fresh Produce
- Avocados, 2
- Beets, 2
- Carrots, 12

- Celery, one head
- Cremini mushrooms, ½ pound
- Garlic, one head
- Ginger, 1 (1-inch) piece
- Leeks, three medium
- Lime, 1
- Mixed berries, two cups
- Portobello mushroom, 1
- Red onions, 2
- Shiitake mushrooms, one and a half pounds
- Sunchokes (Jerusalem artichokes), 4
- Zucchini, three medium
- Apple, 1
- Banana, 1
- Brussels sprouts, ½ pound
- Celeriac (celery root), one medium
- Chard, one bunch
- Escarole, one head
- Garnet yams, 2
- Kale, four bunches
- Lemons, 2
- Mango, 1
- Pear, 1
- Purple cabbage, one small head
- Shallots, 3
- Spinach, 4 cups
- White or yellow onions, two large

Frozen Foods

- Mixed berries, 1 cup
- Butternut squash, 1 cup cubed
- Sweet peas, two cups

Fish, Meat, and Poultry

- Chicken breasts, 2 (4-ounce) boneless and skinless (free-range organic)

- Black cod, 2 pounds
- Lamb sausages, 2
- Whitefish (black cod, cod, or halibut), one and a half pounds
- Salmon, one and a half pounds

Nuts, Seeds, and Dried Fruits

- Almonds, 1 cup raw
- Cashews, one and a quarter cups raw
- Chia seeds, two tablespoons
- Golden raisins, half cup
- Pine nuts, a quarter cup
- Poppy seeds, two teaspoons
- Almond butter, two tablespoons
- Blueberries, half cup freeze-dried
- Cherries, half cup dried
- Dates, half cup pitted
- Mangoes, half cup dried (unsweetened and unsulfured)
- Pistachios, one and a quarter cups shelled
- Pumpkin seeds (pepitas), one and a half cups shelled
- Walnuts, two and a half cups
- Tahini (sesame seed paste), one tablespoon

Herbs and Spices

- Bay leaf, 1
- Celery seed, one teaspoon
- Cinnamon, two tablespoons ground
- Italian herbs, one tablespoon
- Oregano, two tablespoons fresh or one tablespoon dried
- Sage, one teaspoon dried
- Basil leaves, 4 to 5
- Black peppercorns
- Cilantro, one bunch
- Cumin, one teaspoon ground
- Mint, four leaves
- Parsley, one bunch

- Sea salt
- Thyme, two tablespoons fresh or one tablespoon dried
- Sweet paprika, one teaspoon

Oils and Vinegar
- Coconut oil, three tablespoons
- Extra-virgin olive oil, 1 (16-ounce) bottle
- Rice wine vinegar, three tablespoons
- Toasted sesame oil, two tablespoons
- Balsamic vinegar, two tablespoons
- Cooking sherry, two tablespoons
- Flaxseed oil, one tablespoon
- Sunflower oil, two tablespoons

Sweeteners
- Honey, three teaspoons
- Agave nectar, one tablespoon
- Maple syrup (optional), two tablespoons

Other
- Black beans, 1 (15-ounce) can
- Black-eyed peas, one and a half cups dried
- Coconut, half cup unsweetened and shredded
- Green olives, half cup
- Kalamata olives, half cup pitted
- Almond extract, 1/8 teaspoon
- Black lentils, half cup dried
- Coconut milk, half cup unsweetened
- French lentils, half cup dried
- Hemp or almond milk, half cup unsweetened
- Marinated artichoke hearts, 1 (14-ounce) jar
- Vegetable broth, 3 quarts
- Mushroom broth, 1 quart

5.2 Anti-Inflammatory Plate

The trick to a healthy meal plan is finding the best meals on hand and understanding how to eat them in the proper portions. The Anti-Inflammatory Plate will help you maintain track of your portions, and the pantry list will give you the framework you need to build a healthy eating atmosphere. These essential resources help you feed in a way that nourishes and stimulates you without making you feel deprived.

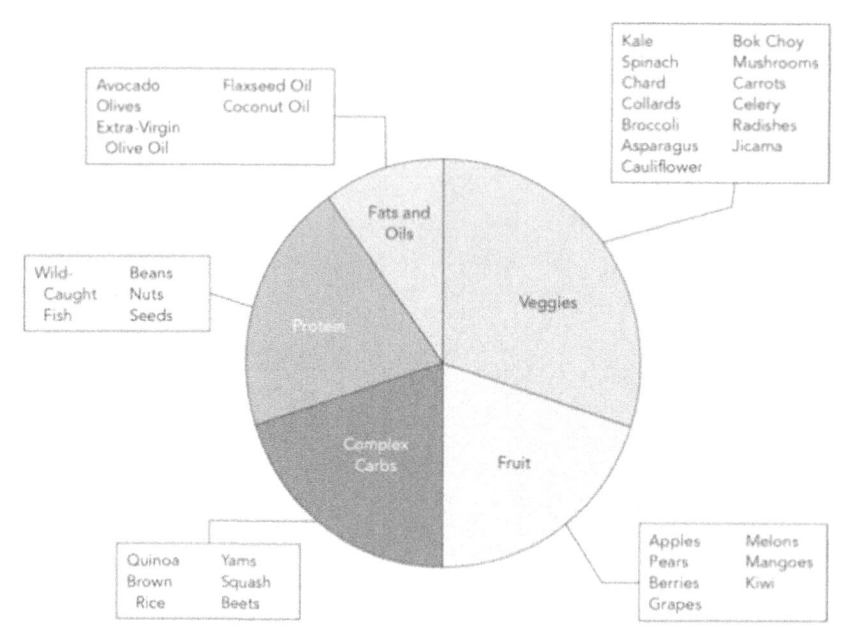

The diagram above illustrates a plate arrangement of food and how you should increase your intake of anti-fighting nutrients to promote health. Forget about the food pyramids from your youth—this Anti-Inflammatory Plate image shows how to eat to enhance your defense against inflammation.

From looking at this chart, you'll find the vegetables take up the majority of the space on the plate. Conjugated linoleic acid (CLA) and other antioxidant vitamins and minerals contained in whole milk are the best for you; in addition, bright, antioxidant-rich fruits have a role to play, as their fiber content tends to reduce the glycaemic index of blood sugar. To begin with, simply aim to increase your daily vegetable intake to two times your current intake of fruits.

While some complex carbohydrates are fruits and vegetables, whole grains, such as brown rice and beets, and quinoa are better sources of carbohydrates, others, such as sweet potatoes and yams, are lower on the glycaemic index and easier to digest, so they're an excellent carbohydrate option as well. Complex carbs are essential for fueling our bodies and for long periods of activity because they provide us with energy and nutrients for extended periods of time. So, soaked yet unrefined, whole grains make for a more substantial meal and have nutrition that is fully used, and black beans make a great with soy. He spoke about the lesser amount of protein that is used on this portion of the plate is somewhat less than on the usual in America. Fish is the safest choice for those who choose to decrease their risk of inflammatory protein, but grass-fed beef, lamb, and poultry are suitable for a few individuals. There are a lot of plant-based protein options that involve legumes, nuts, grains, and soy. Whole soy foods, such as edamame, tempeh, tofu, and miso, can be great additions to a plant-based diet.

This cookbook does not have any hypoallergenic ingredients, which means that soy may not be an issue for those with food allergies; however, of course, soy is one of the most allergenic foods.

In addition, it is essential to remember that there is a section designated for fats and oils on the dish. Obesity is a diet problem that can be replaced by a healthier fat with an anti-inflammatory diet: It's time to get rid of those '80s era fears and eat the nutritious, fulfilling, satiating, and enjoyable ones we ate then. There are large amounts of unsaturated fats and plant oils in this list. This is a list dominated by anti-inflammatory molecules, such as omega-3 and polyunsaturated fats. This diet containing saturated fat will often make you satisfied and usually helps you substantially to curb overindulgence in food.

5.3 The Anti-Inflammatory Pantry

Having ingredients that complement your fitness and wellbeing objectives in your pantry and freezer is a massive move in the right direction. You'll be ready to create anti-inflammatory meals easily if you have the following ingredients on hand, and you'll stop needing to make a memorable trip to the supermarket at the last minute. Since all of the items mentioned can be kept for multiple weeks or longer, you may be able to consume them well before their expiration dates.

MUST-HAVES	BENEFITS	USES	STORAGE
Fats and Oils			
Avocado oil	Great source of monounsaturated fat; more heat stable than olive oil	Frying, sautéing, roasting, grilling; dressings, marinades	Pantry
Coconut oil	Body uses this type of fat as energy; cholesterol-free	Sautéing; butter or shortening replacement	Pantry
Flaxseed oil	Plant-based source of omega-3s	Finishing only (do not heat); dressings, smoothies	Refrigerator
Grapeseed oil	Naturally stable oil that does not oxidize at higher temperatures	Frying, sautéing, roasting, grilling	Pantry
Extra-virgin olive oil	Great source of monounsaturated fat with unique antioxidant polyphenols that have anti-inflammatory properties	Light sautéing, finishing; dressings, marinades	Refrigerator or cool, dark pantry
Nuts and Seeds			
Almonds	Contain healthy fats that decrease inflammation, help lower cholesterol; rich source of vitamin E	Snacking, topping (baked goods, salads, etc.); almond butter, almond milk	Airtight container in pantry
Flaxseeds	Excellent plant-based source of omega-3s; unique forms of fiber that improve digestion	Topping (baked goods, salads, etc.); smoothies; egg replacer	Sealed bag in refrigerator or freezer
Pumpkin seeds	Provide a very diverse blend of antioxidants; good source of magnesium, zinc, iron	Snacking, topping (baked goods, salads, etc.); pumpkin seed butter	Airtight container in pantry
Walnuts	Contains higher amounts of omega-3s than other nuts; rich in anti-inflammatory phytonutrients	Snacking, topping (baked goods, salads, etc.); dips, spreads	Airtight container in refrigerator or cool, dark pantry
Grains and Legumes			
Buckwheat (flour or groats)	Not actually a grain but a very nourishing fruit seed; gluten-free, so a good flour alternative for those avoiding wheat or gluten	Bean or grain dishes, soups, stews, salads; flour replacement	Flour: Sealed bag in freezer; Groats: Pantry
Legumes (adzuki, black, chickpea, lentils, navy, pinto)	Excellent source of fiber, particularly soluble fiber; valuable plant-based source of protein, essential nutrients; gluten-free	Bean or grain dishes, soups, stews, salads, dips	Pantry
Quinoa (flour or whole)	The only grain considered a complete protein; contains small amounts of omega-3s; gluten-free	Bean or grain dishes, soups, stews, salads	Flour: Sealed bag in freezer; Whole: Pantry
Rice (flour or whole: black, brown, purple, red)	Excellent source of fiber, antioxidants that protect against type 2 diabetes and heart disease; gluten-free	Bean or grain dishes, soups, stews, salads	Flour: Sealed bag in freezer; Whole: Pantry

Herbs and Spices				
Cinnamon	Inhibits release of pro-inflammatory messengers in the body; helps regulate blood sugar	Fruit, oatmeal, smoothies, chili, stews	Pantry
Cumin	Stimulates digestive enzymes; contains cancer-preventing compounds	Beans, vegetables, chili, dips, marinades	Pantry
Ginger (dried or fresh)	Contains the anti-inflammatory compounds gingerols; immune-boosting properties	Smoothies, dressings, vegetables, desserts, teas	Dried: Pantry; Fresh: Refrigerator
Oregano (dried or fresh)	Excellent source of vitamin K, which helps regulate the body's inflammatory processes	Beans, vegetables, chili, dips, marinades	Dried: Pantry; Fresh: Refrigerator
Rosemary (dried or fresh)	Contains compounds that stimulate immune system, improve circulation, decrease inflammation	Beans, vegetables, chili, dips, marinades	Dried: Pantry; Fresh: Refrigerator
Turmeric (dried or fresh)	Contains curcumin and volatile oils that have powerful anti-inflammatory effects	Curries, soups, stews, rice, vegetables, lentils	Dried: Pantry; Fresh: Refrigerator

Most people would be able to start returning equilibrium to their bodies and changing their fitness by simply stocking their pantry with the products mentioned here by utilizing the Anti-Inflammatory Plate as a model. Others need a more thorough makeover before they can begin a new nutritional regimen. Although most people feel fine after doing the cleanse, it's especially beneficial for those who have irritable bowel syndrome or intestinal distress, osteo- or rheumatoid arthritis, cough or sinusitis, and skin disorders like eczema or psoriasis. The cleanse is undoubtedly an optional course of action; read the directions carefully and see if it's correct for you. Otherwise, feel free to jump right to the recipes and get cooking!

Chapter 6- 4-Week Meal Plan for an Anti-Inflammatory Diet

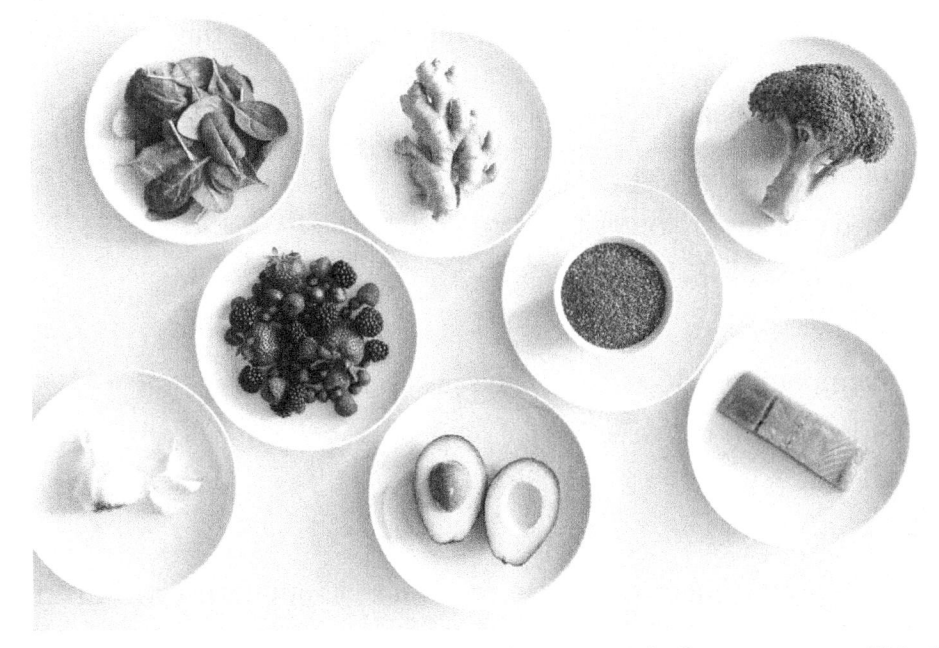

This is the point at which the rubber hits the road. An anti-inflammatory will help you if you've had persistent inflammation for as long as you can recall or if you really want to keep a grip on it until it becomes a challenge. The trick to a successful cleanse is to pair it with nutritionally dense foods that supply the body with the resources it needs to recover. I'm not a fan of juice cleanses or fasting as a way to reduce inflammation in the body. The effects of such cleanse, at most, transient.

By implementing this meal plan, on the other hand, you'll learn how to nourish yourself with whole tasty foods that promote good health. You'll be avoiding ingredients that are frequently linked to inflammation, as well as foods that are in the top eight allergens. If you have an allergic reaction to something you consume on a daily basis, such as pasta, cheese, or eggs, you're unintentionally maintaining an acidic condition in your body.

The elimination diet, which is the gold standard for diagnosing food allergies, is the foundation of the program that is highly prescribed.

In addition to the regular omissions, this schedule requires you to avoid vegetables classified as nightshades, such as potatoes, peppers, tomatoes, and eggplant. Although these things aren't really pro-inflammatory for anyone, they do produce a substance known as alkaloids, which certain people have trouble digesting. I've had a lot of arthritis patients tell me that during tomato season, as they're picking their lovely crops and consuming tomatoes to their hearts' content, their symptoms get dramatically worse.

The natural response to some sort of deprivation diet is to concentrate on the things you can't consume. Many who concentrate most on all of the beautiful, nourishing, anti-inflammatory ingredients that they should consume can see the most significant effects and reap the long-term advantages of this dietary cleanse. The list of foods to add and remove during the cleanse can be found in Phase II, and I've outlined several "best bet" foods that have unique properties that are believed to reduce inflammatory processes in the body. And if all you did was increase the amount of these best-bet items in your regular diet, you're sure to see a good change in yourself.

6.1 Helpful Advises and Suggestions to Get Started

In brief, no matter which anti-inflammatory diet you use, below are the specific recommendations to follow:

1. Eat a wide variety of fruits and vegetables.
2. Consume fats that are safe for you.
3. Achieve a balanced omega-6 to omega-3 ratio.
4. Get enough protein in your diet.
5. Help and cure the gut.
6. Restrict the consumption of added sugars and processed foods.
7. Per day, drink at least eight glasses of water.
8. Take care of the stress rate.
9. Have a good night's sleep.

With these considerations in mind, it's time to read more about each anti-inflammatory strategy and choose the best one for you.

6.2 Phase One – The Preparation

The planning process is the first step in starting an anti-inflammatory diet. First, take a peek at your calendar and locate a one-month span free of travel or social obligations—this is the best way to work a cleanse into your schedule with the best results. Then it's time to begin the cleansing preparations. Before you start, I usually suggest allowing yourself a week to prepare your body and pantry. For specific individuals, giving up coffee and sugar is one of the most challenging aspects of this cleanse, but use this planning week to help alleviate dependency, which can reduce painful withdrawal symptoms.

Caffeine intake should be reduced

Begin weaning yourself off caffeine now, whether you're using it in some way. If you drink coffee, gradually reduce the caffeine content to half-decaf, absolute decaf (preferably Swiss Water decaf), green or black tea, and finally, herbal tea. Switch to caffeine-free sodas and only substitute with water if you consume soda. Reduce the amount of caffeine you consume per day before you've finally eliminated it from your diet.

Some weaning suggestions

Reduce the caffeine intake by 25% over the first two days, then drink two more glasses of water per day. In the third and fourth days, reduce caffeine intake by another 25% while managing to consume plenty of water. On the fifth day, cut out all caffeine and replace it with herbal tea and water.

Avoid adding sugar to your diet or drinks, and steer clear of refined foods with sugar mentioned among the first five ingredients.

Have an appointment for a massage or treatment to assist with depression and other withdrawal symptoms.

Allow yourself some time throughout the week to adapt to these adjustments, and be aware that minor withdrawal symptoms and brain fog can occur. If you're having trouble concentrating, it may be beneficial to take a day or two off work.

Begin Water to drink

Start by rising your water consumption to at least sixty to seventy ounces of water or herbal tea a day.

This helps you wash away contaminants while still keeping you hydrated and will assist with withdrawal symptoms.

Let the Sugar Beast be under control

Reduce your intake of added sugar and begin reviewing the nutrient labeling and ingredient lists on all processed foods you purchase, and develop the habit of learning precisely what's in your diet. Products containing starch, sucrose, evaporated cane juice, high fructose corn syrup, or chemical sweeteners like sucralose or aspartame should be avoided.

Stock up on the Essentials

Fruits, beans, vegetables, brown rice or quinoa, seeds, nuts, and fish can all be on the shopping list.

Your Metabolism Has to Be Revved Up

Make it a routine to consume a good breakfast within an hour of waking up, and then a quick lunch or healthy snack every three or four hours.

Put the best foot forward

Have a food schedule and a grocery list for the first week after the cleanse. It's a brilliant idea to have a well-stocked pantry and refrigerator, as well as to do some meal planning ahead of time, such as washing and slicing tomatoes, preparing a sandwich, and cooking quinoa or rice. Spending a couple of hours ahead of time can allow the cleanse much more fun, as well as keep you stress-free and on schedule. Finally, prepare to be blown away.

6.3 Phase Two- The Nourishment and Cleansing

The nourishment and cleansing process is the next step.

The top eight allergens (soy, dairy, eggs, peanuts, corn, shellfish, wheat/gluten, and oranges) will be totally eliminated from your diet during this process. Additionally, you can abstain from sugar, caffeine, and alcohol. If you have knee inflammation or an overt inflammatory disorder (such as inflammatory bowel disease), you should avoid nightshade vegetables (eggplant, tomatoes, potatoes, and peppers) to see if the alkaloid-rich foods are aggravating the symptoms.

So, what are your options? What's left is a Mediterranean-style diet that's both nutritious and anti-inflammatory. Vegetables, nuts, fruits, seeds, gluten-free whole grains, legumes, finfish, and limited quantities of healthy meat and poultry can be the primary sources of nutrition.

If you prepare ahead, you will not go hungry.

The best foods include phytonutrients and essential fatty acids, which help your body reverse inflammatory processes. These are the items you can want to consume more often, with the aim of having at least five of them in your diet on a daily basis.

	FOODS TO INCLUDE	BEST BETS	FOODS TO EXCLUDE
Vegetables	Fresh raw, steamed, sautéed, juiced, or roasted vegetables	Beets, broccoli, brussels sprouts, carrots, chard, kale, onions, spinach, garnet or jewel yams	Corn, creamed vegetables, nightshades (eggplant, peppers, potatoes, tomatoes)
Fruits	Fresh or frozen fruits, unsweetened fruit juices	Apples, avocados, berries, grapes, kiwis, melons, pears	Oranges, orange juice
Grains	Amaranth, buckwheat, millet, oats (certified gluten-free), quinoa, rice, tapioca, teff	Buckwheat, quinoa, rice (brown or red)	Barley, corn, gluten-containing products, kamut, rye, spelt, wheat
Animal Proteins: Fish and Meat	Fresh, frozen, or canned (water-packed) fish; small amounts of 100% grass-fed beef, wild game, lamb, free-range organic poultry	Wild-caught finfish: black cod, cod, halibut, salmon, sardines	Canned meats, cold cuts, eggs, frankfurters, pork, sausage, shellfish
Vegetable Proteins: Legumes	All beans (except soy), peas, lentils	Adzuki beans, black-eyed peas, hummus, lentils, mung beans	All soy products, including edamame, soy milk, tempeh, tofu
Fats	Almond, coconut, flaxseed, grapeseed, extra-virgin olive, pumpkin, safflower, sunflower, sesame, and walnut oils	Coconut oil, grapeseed oil, extra-virgin olive oil, olives	Butter, margarine, mayonnaise, processed and hydrogenated oils, shortening, spreads
Nuts and Seeds	Almonds, cashews, walnuts; chia, pumpkin, sesame, and sunflower seeds; butters made from these nuts and seeds, tahini	Almonds, chia seeds, pumpkin seeds, walnuts	Peanuts, peanut butter
Spices, Condiments, and Confections	All spices, vinegar, mustard (grain-free, made from mustard seed and vinegar)	Cinnamon, garlic, ginger, oregano, rosemary, turmeric	Barbecue sauce, chocolate and chocolate sauce, chutney, cocoa, ketchup, relish, soy sauce, other condiments
Dairy and Milk Substitutes	Unsweetened almond, coconut, hemp, rice, and other nut or seed milks	Unsweetened almond, coconut, and hemp milks	Butter, cheese, cottage cheese, cow's milk, cream, frozen yogurt, ice cream, yogurt
Beverages	Filtered or distilled water, herbal tea, seltzer or mineral water	Herbal tea, water	Alcohol, coffee, all caffeinated and/or sweetened beverages
Sweeteners	Agave nectar, blackstrap molasses, coconut palm sugar, fruit sweetener, honey, pure maple syrup, stevia	Blackstrap molasses, coconut palm sugar, raw honey	Aspartame, corn syrup, evaporated cane juice, high-fructose corn syrup, refined sugar (white or brown), sucralose, other artificial sweeteners

6.4 Phase Three- The Reintroduction

You might feel so amazing after weeks of clean eating and blissful nourishment that you don't want to alter a thing. Although it's encouraging that you're already excited about healthier eating when you near the end of the cleanse, keep in mind that some of the things you avoided during Phase II are completely acceptable alternatives. Let's look at soy as an example: Whole soy foods like tempeh, tofu, and edamame may be a perfect way to get calcium, protein, and a variety of other phytonutrients if you absorb them well and decide to consume a more plant-based diet.

During the third phase, you have a few choices for reintroducing foods. You have the option of doing a less organized, gradual reintroduction of the foods you've been missing or doing more formal diet challenges. The latter is intended for those who suspect they have severe food allergies or intolerances. When anyone has serious stomach problems or skin problems that go away after a cleanse, I usually recommend that they do structured diet reintroductions and figure out which food or foods are triggering the symptoms.

Whatever choice you chose, bear in mind that you want to build on your progress and maintain some of the good habits you've developed. You just don't want to shock the brain by inadvertently exposing it to anything you've been ignoring with one fell swoop. Celebrating the completion of a cleanse with a big meat pie, a pitcher of soda, and an ice cream sundae is usually not a pleasant idea.

Option 1: Slowly reintroduce the foods (Less Structured)

1. Reintroduce foods gradually while maintaining balanced eating patterns (such as eating more vegetables and fresh, whole foods).
2. Try to stick to one new food category every day while reintroducing foods, and hold portion sizes in check (e.g., challenge dairy by having some plain yogurt with fruit and see how that goes).
3. Keep a diary and keep track of the shifts in your mood when you reintroduce foods into your diet. This can help you draw the dots if there are any foods that aggravate the system in any way.

Option 2: Formal Food Reintroductions (More Structured)

1. Primarily choose the food category to reintroduce:

- Eggs
- Wheat/gluten
- Corn
- Citrus
- Dairy
- Soy
- Peanuts
- Nightshades (eggplant, peppers, potatoes, tomatoes)
- Optional: Caffeine, sugar, and alcohol (challenge certain drugs to see how susceptible you are, so it's only reasonable to practice to enjoy them in moderation, if at all) are optional.

2. During the course of one day, consume two to three average-size portions of a pure type of food from that category. A pure type indicates that the meal should not have any chemicals or other products that you have been avoiding (e.g., sugar).

Here are several samples of pure foods from various groups:

- Wheat/gluten—Whole wheat tortilla, whole wheat pasta
- Dairy—Milk, plain yogurt, and cheese with no artificial color or taste.
- Soy- Edamame, tempeh and pure soy milk are all made from

3. Eliminate the food category from the diet after one day of feeding on it. Regardless of how you respond, you can hold this food category out of your diet before the conclusion of the reintroduction process. Keep track of how you're doing over two days, giving you enough flexibility to notice both sudden and delayed reactions. Use a journal or folder to keep track of the foods you're introducing and any possible reactions—write about anything that's changed from when you were in the diet's complete elimination phase.

Examples of possible reactions are as under: -

- Gas, bloating, or discomfort in the abdomen
- Pain Anxiety, exhaustion, or fatigue
- Skin irritations or breakouts
- Constipation or diarrhea
- Pressure in the muscles or joints

4. Reintroduce the next food category if you don't have any effects within two days. Remember that you are challenging each food category separately because even though you have no response, delete the food group from your diet after testing it before you've finished all food reintroductions. If you have symptoms after challenging a meal, avoid eating it and wait for the symptoms to subside before moving on to the next task.
5. For each food group, repeat steps two through four.

6.5 Phase Four - Transition to Long-Term Anti-Inflammatory Eating

Once you've finished your nutrient cleanse and progressed through the diet reintroductions, you'll want to determine which routines are worth keeping, ideally for the rest of your existence. I still like to tell you that it isn't a quick fix or a "Hollywood cleanse." The aim is to align your body and continue on the road to health. If you catch yourself in a hurry to reintroduce any of your beloved inflammatory ingredients (processed, sugary snacks, or so much meat), remind yourself of all the ways a clean diet has helped you: more stamina, a shift of body shape, reduced achiness and joint discomfort, a glowing skin, and so on.

Here are few pointers to get you on track during your cleanse:

1. Have a weekly or monthly meal plan—healthy eating isn't something that happens by accident!
2. Take Michael Pollan's advice and do the following: "Eat some food. Most of the items are plants. "Don't go overboard."
3. Consume two times the amounts of fruits and vegetables.
4. Tame the sugar. (primarily by avoiding refined sugar).
5. Stop heavily refined wheat goods when opting for whole grains.
6. Pack your own lunches and treats to reduce your intake of packaged foods.
7. Find pleasure in the very movement! Exercising can be pleasant.
8. Every day, take a few minutes to breathe, calm and regroup.
9. Make a bedtime routine and try to get seven to nine hours of sleep each night.
10. Be polite, compassionate, and caring to yourself. It's not quick to alter!

6.6 Meal Plan

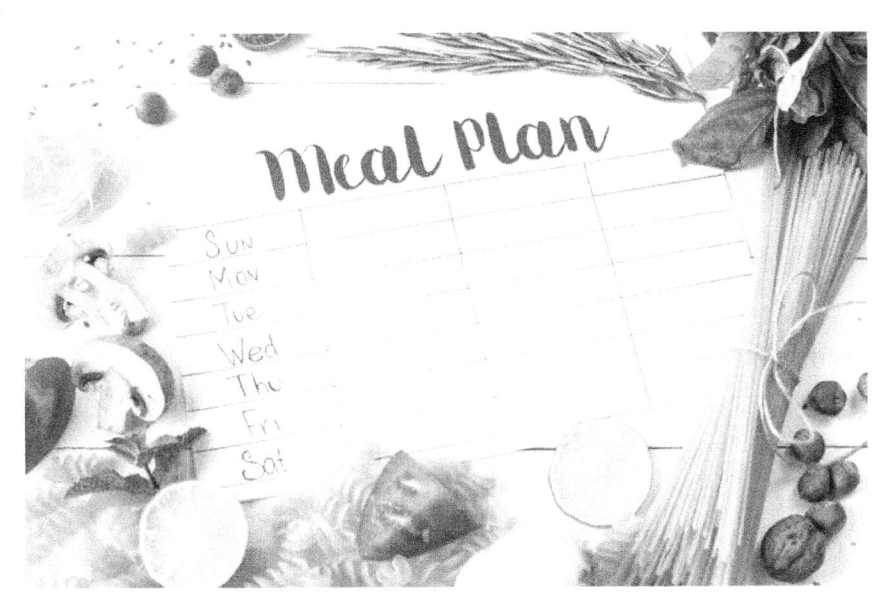

1st Week

Day 1

Breakfast- Cherry Smoothie

Snack-Sweet Potato Chips

Lunch-Chicken stir-fry

Snack-Half an apple

Dinner-Black bean Chili with Garlic and Tomatoes

Day 2

Breakfast- Spinach Frittata

Snack-Mango-Thyme Smoothie

Lunch-Shrimp Scampi

Snack-Half an avocado

Dinner-Buckwheat Noodles with Peanut Sauce

Day 3

Breakfast-Buckwheat Crepes with Berries

Snack-One banana

Lunch-Soba Noodle Soup with Spinach

Snack-Kale chips

Dinner-Roasted salmon and asparagus

Day 4

Breakfast- Green Apple Smoothie

Snack-Sweet potato Chips

Lunch-Fried rice with kale

Snack-Mini snack muffin

Dinner-Chicken cacciatore

Day 5

Breakfast-Sweet Potato Hash

Snack-Green Apple smoothie

Lunch-Pork chops with Gingered Applesauce

Snack-Anti-inflammatory Trail Mix

Dinner-Sweet Potato Curry with Spinach

Day 6

Breakfast-Green Smoothie

Snack-Smoked Trout and Mango Wraps

Lunch-Squash and Ginger Soup

Snack-Herbal tea

Dinner-Rosemary Chicken

Day 7

Breakfast- Mushroom and bell pepper Parfait

Snack-Kale and Banana Smoothie

Lunch-Quinoa Florentine

Snack-Kale Chips

Dinner-Turkey with Bell Peppers and Rosemary

2nd Week

Day 1

Breakfast-Chai Smoothie

Snack-Mashed Avocado with Jicama Slices

Lunch-Beef and Broccoli Stir-Fry

Snack-Gluten-free Oat and Fruit Bars

Dinner-Mushroom Pesto Burgers

Day 2

Breakfast- Chia Breakfast Pudding

Snack-Crunchy Spicy Chickpeas

Lunch-Tomato Asparagus Frittata

Snack-Mashed Avocado with Jicama Slices

Dinner-Beef Tenderloin with Savory Blueberry Sauce

Day 3

Breakfast- Mushroom and bell pepper Parfait

Snack-Super Green Smoothie

Lunch-Shrimp with Cinnamon Sauce

Snack-Nutty Coconut Energy Truffle

Dinner- Whole-Wheat Pasta with Tomato-Basil Sauce

Day 4

Breakfast-Coconut Pancakes

Snack-Cherry Smoothie

Lunch-Turkey Scaloppine with Rosemary and Lemon Sauce

Snack-Frozen Berries

Dinner-Rosemary Chicken

Day 5

Breakfast-Ginger-Berry Smoothie

Snack-Sweet Potato Chips

Lunch-Citrus Salmon on a Bed of Greens

Snack-Herbal tea

Dinner-Chicken and Bell pepper Sauté

Day 6

Breakfast-Mango Muesli with Brazil nut topping

Snack- Half an apple

Lunch-Tuscan Chicken

Snack-Tropical Quinoa Power Bars

Dinner-Tofu and Spinach Sauté

Day 7

Breakfast- Buckwheat Crepes with Berries

Snack- Crunchy Spicy Chickpeas

Lunch-Easy Chicken and Broccoli

Snack-Kale Chips

Dinner-Cod with Ginger and Black Beans

3rd Week

Day 1

Breakfast- Spinach Frittata

Snack-Half an apple

Lunch-Ground Turkey and Spinach Stir-Fry

Snack-Blueberry Nut Trail Mix

Dinner-Orange and Maple-Glazed Salmon

Day 2

Breakfast-Mushroom frittata

Snack-Blueberry, Chocolate, and Turmeric Smoothie

Lunch-Macadamia-Dusted Pork Cutlets

Snack-Frozen berries

Dinner-Whole-wheat Pasta with Tomato-Basil Sauce

Day 3

Breakfast- Mushroom and bell pepper Parfait

Snack- Crunchy Spicy Chickpeas

Lunch-Salmon Ceviche

Snack-Herbal Tea

Dinner-Pan- Seared Scallops with Lemon-Ginger Vinaigrette

Day 4

Breakfast-Sweet and Savory Quinoa Crepes

Snack-Protein Powerhouse Smoothie

Lunch-Manhattan-Style Salmon Chowder

Snack-Strawberry-chia Ice Pops

Dinner-Beef Tenderloin with Savory Blueberry Sauce

Day 5

Breakfast- Spinach Frittata

Snack-Coconut-Ginger Smoothie

Lunch-Lamb Meatballs with Garlic Aioli

Snack- Shiitake Mushrooms and Walnut Pate

Dinner-Black Bean Chili with Garlic and Tomatoes

Day 6

Breakfast- Overnight Muesli

Snack-Berry Green Power Smoothie

Lunch-Quinoa-Stuffed Collard Rolls

Snack-Tropical Quinoa Power Bars

Dinner-Thin-cut Pork Chops with Mustardy Kale

Day 7

Breakfast-Kale and Banana Smoothie

Snack-Mini Snack Muffins

Lunch-Tofu Sloppy Joes

Snack-Blueberry Nut Trail Mix

Dinner-Halibut Curry

4th Week

Day 1

Breakfast-Spinach Muffins

Snack-Green Apple Smoothie

Lunch-Turkey-Burgers with Ginger-Teriyaki Sauce and Pineapple

Snack-Anti-inflammatory Trail Mix

Dinner-Mustard and Rosemary Pork Tenderloin

Day 2

Breakfast- Mushroom and bell pepper Parfait

Snack-Half an apple

Lunch-Chicken Stir -fry

Snack- Shiitake Mushrooms and Walnut Pate

Dinner-Fish Taco Salad with Strawberry Avocado Salsa

Day 3

Breakfast- Overnight Muesli

Snack- Crunchy Spicy Chickpeas

Lunch-Beef and Bell Pepper Fajitas

Snack-Strawberry-Chia Ice Pops

Dinner-Veggie Pizza with Cauliflower-Yam Crust

Day 4

Breakfast-Spinach Frittata

Snack-Half an avocado

Lunch-Chicken Adobo

Snack-Shiitake Mushrooms and Walnut Pate

Dinner-Beef and Bell Pepper Stir-Fry

Day 5

Breakfast- Mushroom and bell pepper Parfait

Snack-Sweet Potato Chips

Lunch-Rosemary-Lemon Cod

Snack-Nutty Coconut Energy Truffle

Dinner-Gingered Turkey Meatballs

Day 6

Breakfast-Coconut Pancakes

Snack-Mashed Avocado with Jicama Slices

Lunch-Fried Rice with Kale

Snack-Herbal Tea

Dinner-Chicken salad Sandwiches

Day 7

Breakfast-Overnight Muesli

Snack-Half an apple

Lunch-Beef Flank Steak Tacos with Guacamole

Snack-Tropical Quinoa Power Bars

Dinner-Toasted Pecan Quinoa Burgers

The list of food provided is not exhaustive in nature. An anti-inflammatory diet is not related to calorie intake but is dependent on the foods that keep your gut healthy. Therefore, you can adjust your meal as per your liking that suits your health the best.

In the upcoming chapters, various recipes are provided for you to try whilst following the anti-inflammatory diet. You need not compromise with your taste buds while being on a diet. The recipes provided are simple and without any lengthy and complex steps.

Chapter 7-Breakfast Recipes

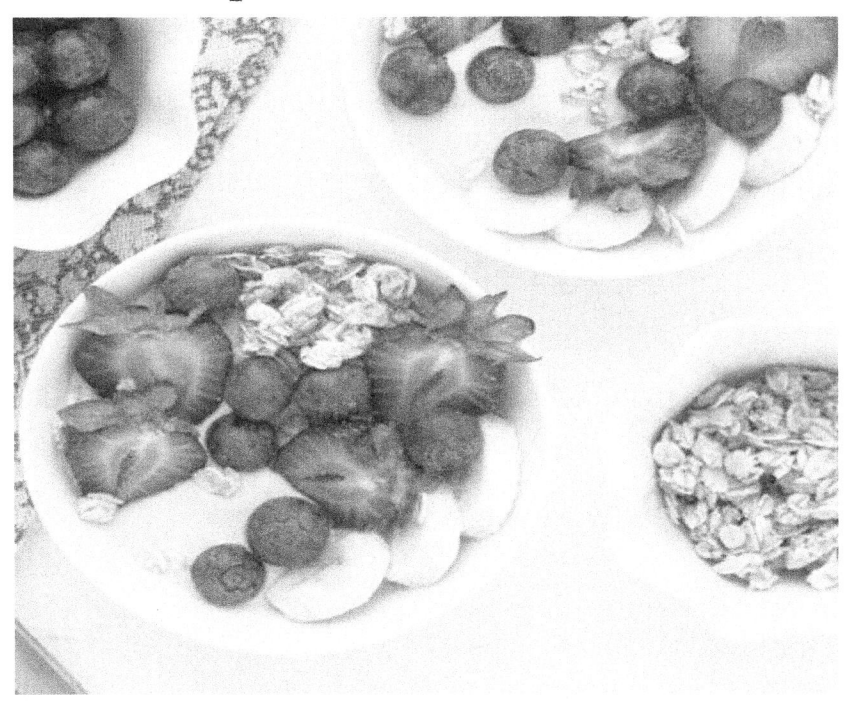

7.1 Spinach Frittata

Preparation time-10 minutes| Cook time-12 minutes| Total time-22 minutes| Servings-2|Difficulty-Easy

Nutritional Facts- Calories: 203; Total Fat: 17g; Total Carbs: 2g; Sugar: <1g; Fiber: <1g; Protein: 13g; Sodium: 402mg

Ingredients

- Two cups of baby spinach
- One teaspoon of garlic powder
- Two tablespoons of extra-virgin olive oil
- Eight beaten eggs
- Half teaspoon of sea salt
- Two tablespoons of grated parmesan cheese
- 1/8 teaspoon of freshly ground black pepper

Instructions

1. Preheat the broiler to the highest setting.
2. Heat the olive oil in a big ovenproof skillet or pan (well-seasoned cast iron fits well) over medium-high heat until it starts shimmering.
3. Cook, stirring regularly, for around 3 minutes after introducing the spinach.
4. Whisk together the eggs, salt, garlic powder, and pepper in a medium mixing cup. Carefully spill the egg mixture over the spinach and cook for 3 minutes, or until the edges of the eggs begin to set.

5. Gently raise the eggs away from the pan's sides with a rubber spatula. Enable the uncooked egg to flow into the pan's edges by tilting it. Cook for another 2 or 3 minutes, just until the sides are solid.
6. Place the pan under the broiler and cover with the Parmesan cheese. Preheat the oven to broil for around 3 minutes, or before the top puffs up.
7. To eat, break into wedges.

7.2 Mushroom and Bell Pepper Omelet

Preparation time-10 minutes| Cook time-10 minutes| Total time-20 minutes| Servings-2|Difficulty-Easy

Nutritional Facts- Calories: 336; Total Fat: 27g; Total Carbs: 7g; Sugar: 5g; Fiber: 1g; Protein: 18g; Sodium: 656mg

Ingredients

- One sliced red bell pepper
- Six beaten eggs
- 1/8 teaspoon of freshly ground black pepper
- Two tablespoons of extra virgin olive oil
- One cup of sliced mushrooms
- Half a teaspoon of sea salt

Instructions

1. Heat the olive oil in a broad non-stick pan over medium heat until it shimmers.
2. Combine the mushrooms and red bell pepper in a mixing dish. Cook, stirring regularly, for around 4 minutes, or until tender.
3. Whisk together the salt, eggs, and pepper in a medium mixing cup. Pour the eggs over the vegetables and cook for around 3 minutes, or until the edges of the eggs begin to set.
4. Gently raise the eggs away from the pan's sides with a rubber spatula. Allow the uncooked egg to flow to the pan's edges by tilting it. Cook for 2 to 3 minutes, or until the edges and core of the eggs are set.
5. Fold the omelet in half with a spatula. To eat, break into wedges.

7.3 Yogurt, Berry, and Walnut Parfait

Preparation time-10 minutes| Cook time-0 minutes| Total time-10 minutes| Servings-2|Difficulty-Easy

Nutritional Facts- Calories: 505; Total Fat: 22g; Total Carbs: 56g; Sugar: 45g; Fiber: 8g; Protein: 23g; Sodium: 174mg

Ingredients

- Two tablespoons of honey
- Two cups of Plain unsweetened coconut yogurt or plain unsweetened yogurt or almond yogurt
- One cup of fresh blueberries

- Half cup of walnut pieces
- One cup of fresh raspberries

Instructions

1. Stir the yogurt and honey together. Divide into two bowls
2. Sprinkle in blueberries and raspberries along with A quarter cup of chopped walnuts

7.4 Oatmeal and Cinnamon with Dried Cranberries

Preparation time-5 minutes| Cook time-8 minutes| Total time-13 minutes| Servings-2|Difficulty-Easy

Nutritional Facts- Calories: 101; Total Fat: 2g; Total Carbs: 18g; Sugar: 1g; Fiber: 4g; Protein: 3g; Sodium: 126mg

Ingredients

- One cup of almond milk
- One cup of oats
- One teaspoon of ground cinnamon
- One cup of water
- One pinch of sea salt
- Half cup of dried cranberries

Instructions

1. Get the almond milk, salt, and water to a boil in a medium saucepan.
2. Stir in the cranberries, oats, and cinnamon. Reduce the heat and stir for 5 minutes.
3. Remove the oats from heat. Allow the pot to stand for 3 minutes. Mix before serving.

7.5 Green Tea and Ginger Shake

Preparation time-5 minutes| Cook time-0 minutes| Total time-5 minutes| Servings-2|Difficulty-Easy

Nutritional Facts- Calories: 340; Total Fat: 7g; Total Carbs: 56g; Sugar: 50g; Fiber: 2g; Protein: 11g; Sodium: 186mg

Ingredients

- Two tablespoons of honey
- Two tablespoons of grated ginger
- Two tablespoons of matcha (green tea) powder
- Two cups of skim milk
- Two scoops of Low-fat Vanilla ice cream

Instructions

1. In a blender, combine all the ingredients and blend until smooth.

7.6 Smoked Salmon Scrambled Eggs

Preparation time-5 minutes| Cook time-8 minutes| Total time-13 minutes| Servings-2|Difficulty-Easy

Nutritional Facts- Calories: 236; Total Fat: 18g; Total Carbs: <1g; Sugar: <1g; Fiber: 0g; Protein: 19g; Sodium: 974mg

Ingredients

- Three ounces of flaked smoked salmon
- Half teaspoon of freshly ground black pepper
- ¾ tablespoon of extra-virgin olive oil
- Four beaten eggs

Instructions

1. Heat the olive oil in a big skillet or pan over medium-high heat until it starts shimmering.
2. Cook for around 3 minutes, stirring occasionally.
3. Beat the eggs and pepper together in a medium mixing cup. Add them to the skillet or pan and cook, stirring gently, for around 5 minutes, or until cooked.

7.7 Chia Breakfast Pudding

Preparation time-10 minutes| Rest time-15 minutes| Total time-25 minutes| Servings-2|Difficulty-Easy

Nutritional Facts- Calories: 272; Total Fat: 14g; Total Carbohydrates: 38g; Sugar: 25g; Fiber: 6g; Protein: 7g; Sodium: 84mg

Ingredients

- Half cup of chia seeds
- Half teaspoon of vanilla extract
- Half cup of chopped cashews, divided
- One cup of almond milk
- A quarter cup of maple syrup or raw honey
- Half cup of frozen no-added-sugar pitted cherries, thawed, juice reserved, divided

Instructions

1. Combine the chia seeds, almond milk, maple syrup, and vanilla in a quart container with a tight-fitting seal. Set aside for at least 15 minutes after thoroughly shaking.
2. Pour the pudding into two bowls and finish with a quarter cup of cherries and two tablespoons of cashews in each.

7.8 Coconut Rice with Berries

Preparation time-10 minutes| Cook time-30 minutes| Total time-40 minutes| Servings-2|Difficulty-Moderate

Nutritional Facts- Calories: 281; Total Fat: 8g; Total Carbohydrates: 49g; Sugar: 7g; Fiber: 5g; Protein: 6g; Sodium: 623mg

Ingredients

- 3/4 cup of water
- 3/4 teaspoon of salt
- Half cup of fresh blueberries, or raspberries, divided
- Half cup of shaved coconut, divided
- Half cup of brown basmati rice
- Half cup of coconut milk
- Two pitted and chopped dates
- A quarter cup of toasted slivered almonds, divided

Instructions

1. Combine the water, basmati rice, coconut milk, spice, and date pieces in a medium saucepan over high heat.
2. Stir constantly until the mixture boils. Reduce the heat to low and cook, occasionally stirring, for 20 to 30 minutes, or until the rice is tender.
3. Place some blueberries, almonds, and coconut on top of each serving of rice.

7.9 Overnight Muesli

Preparation time-10 minutes| Cook time-0 minutes| Total time-10 minutes| Servings-2|Difficulty-Easy

Nutritional Facts- Calories: 213; Total Fat: 4g; Total Carbohydrates: 39g; Sugar: 10g; Fiber: 6g; Protein: 6g; Sodium: 74mg

Ingredients

- One cup of gluten-free rolled oats
- One cup of coconut milk
- A quarter cup of no-added-sugar apple juice
- One tablespoon of apple cider vinegar (optional)
- Half cored and chopped apple
- Dash ground cinnamon

Instructions

1. Combine the oats, apple juice, coconut milk, and vinegar in a medium mixing dish.
2. Refrigerate overnight, covered.
3. The following day, add the sliced apple and a pinch of cinnamon to the muesli.

7.10 Spicy Quinoa

Preparation time-10 minutes| Cook time-20 minutes| Total time-30 minutes| Servings-2|Difficulty-Easy

Nutritional Facts- Calories: 286; Total Fat: 13g; Total Carbohydrates: 32g; Sugar: 1g; Fiber: 6g; Protein: 10g; Sodium: 44mg

Ingredients

- One cup of water
- A quarter cup of hemp seeds
- Half teaspoon of ground cinnamon
- Pinch salt
- A quarter cup of chopped hazelnuts
- Half cup of quinoa rinsed well
- A quarter cup of shredded coconut
- One tablespoon of flaxseed
- Half teaspoon of vanilla extract
- Half cup of fresh berries of your choice, divided

Instructions

1. Combine the quinoa and water in a medium saucepan over high heat.
2. Bring to a boil, then reduce to low heat and continue to cook for 15 to 20 minutes, or until the quinoa is tender.
3. Combine the coconut, flaxseed, hemp seeds, cinnamon, vanilla, and salt in a large mixing bowl.
4. Divide the quinoa into two bowls and finish with some berries and hazelnuts for each serving.

7.11 Buckwheat Crêpes with Berries

Preparation time-15 minutes| Cook time-5 minutes per crepe| Total time-40 minutes| Servings-2|Difficulty-Moderate

Nutritional Facts- Calories: 242; Total Fat: 11g; Total Carbohydrates: 33g; Sugar: 9g; Fiber: 6g; Protein: 7g; Sodium: 371mg

Ingredients

- Half teaspoon of salt
- One cup of almond milk or water
- Half teaspoon of vanilla extract
- Three tablespoons of Chia Jam
- Half cup of buckwheat flour
- One tablespoon of coconut oil (Half tablespoon melted)
- One egg

- Two cups of fresh berries, divided

Instructions

1. Whisk together the salt, egg, buckwheat flour, and half tablespoon melted coconut oil, almond milk, and vanilla in a small mixing bowl until smooth.
2. Melt the remaining half tablespoon of coconut oil in a wide (12-inch) non-stick skillet or pan over medium-high heat. Tilt the pan to adequately cover it in the molten oil.
3. Using a ladle in the skillet or pan, pour half a cup of batter. Tilt the pan to properly brush it with batter.
4. Cook for another 2 minutes, or until the edges start to curl. Flip the crêpe with a spatula and cook for 1 minute on the other hand. Place the crêpe on a plate and set aside.
5. For the left batter, continue to make crêpe.
6. On a dish, place one crêpe, some berries, and a tablespoon of Chia Jam. Fold the crêpe over the filling and seal the edges.

7.12 Warm Chia-Berry Non-dairy Yogurt

Preparation time-10 minutes| Cook time-5 minutes| Total time-15 minutes| Servings-2|Difficulty-Easy

Nutritional Facts- Calories: 246; Total Fat: 10g; Total Carbohydrates: 35g; Sugar: 21g; Fiber: 5g; Protein: 5g; Sodium: 2mg

Ingredients

- One tablespoon of maple syrup
- Half vanilla bean halved lengthwise
- Two cups of unsweetened almond yogurt or coconut yogurt
- One (10-ounce) package frozen mixed berries, thawed
- One tablespoon of freshly squeezed lemon juice
- Half tablespoon of chia seeds

Instructions

1. Combine the berries, lemon juice, maple syrup, and vanilla bean in a medium saucepan over medium-high flame.
2. Get the mixture to a boil, continuously stirring. Reduce the heat to low heat and continue to cook for 3 minutes.
3. Switch off the heat from the pan. Remove the vanilla bean from the mixture and discard it. Add the chia seeds and mix well. Allow 5 to 10 minutes for the seeds to thicken.
4. Cover each bowl with one cup of yogurt and divide the fruit mixture among both of them.

7.13 Buckwheat Waffles

Preparation time-15 minutes| Cook time-6 minutes per waffle| Total time-40 minutes| Servings-2|Difficulty-Moderate

Nutritional Facts- Calories: 282; Total Fat: 4g; Total Carbohydrates: 55g; Sugar: 7g; Fiber: 6g; Protein: 9g; Sodium: 692mg

Ingredients

- Half cup of brown rice flour
- Half teaspoon of baking soda
- One egg
- One cup of buckwheat flour
- One teaspoon of baking powder
- Half teaspoon of salt
- One tablespoon of maple syrup
- Half cup of water
- One cup of almond milk
- Coconut oil for the waffle iron
- One teaspoon of vanilla extract

Instructions

1. Whisk together the buckwheat flour, baking powder, rice flour, baking soda, and salt in a medium mixing dish.
2. Add the maple syrup, egg, and vanilla to the dry ingredients. Whisk in the water and almond milk in a slow, steady stream until smooth.
3. The batter is absolutely free of lumps.
4. Allow 10 minutes for the batter to thicken slightly.
5. When the buckwheat is resting, it can settle to the bottom of the dish, so stir thoroughly before using.
6. Brush the waffle iron with coconut oil and heat it.
7. In the waffle iron, pour the batter and cook according to the manufacturer's instructions.

7.14 Coconut Pancakes

Preparation time-10 minutes| Cook time-5 minutes per pancake| Total time-20 minutes| Servings-2|Difficulty-Easy

Nutritional Facts- Calories: 193; Total Fat: 11g; Total Carbohydrates: 15g; Sugar: 6g; Fiber: 6g; Protein: 9g; Sodium: 737mg

Ingredients

- Half cup of coconut or almond milk, plus additional as needed
- Half tablespoon of maple syrup
- A quarter cup of coconut flour
- Half teaspoon of salt

- Two eggs
- Half tablespoon of melted coconut oil or almond butter, plus additional for greasing the pan
- Half teaspoon of vanilla extract
- Half teaspoon of baking soda

Instructions

1. Using an electric mixer, combine the coconut milk, maple syrup, eggs, coconut oil, and vanilla in a medium mixing cup.
2. Combine the baking soda, coconut flour, and salt in a shallow mixing bowl. Combine the dry ingredients with the wet ingredients in a mixing bowl and beat until smooth and lump-free.
3. If the batter is too dense, add more liquid to thin it down to a typical pancake batter consistency.
4. Using coconut oil, lightly grease a big skillet or pan. Preheat the oven to medium-high.
5. Cook for around 3 minutes, or until golden brown on the rim. Cook for another 2 minutes on the other hand.
6. Continue to cook the leftover batter while stacking the pancake on a tray.

7.15 Spinach Muffins

Preparation time-15 minutes| Cook time-15 minutes| Total time-30 minutes| Servings-6 muffins| Difficulty-Moderate

Nutritional Facts- Calories: 108; Total Fat: 6g; Total Carbohydrates: 12g; Sugar: 6g; Fiber: 1g; Protein: 3g; Sodium: 217mg

Ingredients

- One cup of packed spinach
- A quarter cup of raw honey
- Half teaspoon of vanilla extract
- Half cup of almond flour
- Half teaspoon of baking soda
- Pinch freshly ground black pepper
- Cooking spray
- One egg
- Two tablespoons of extra-virgin olive oil
- Half cup of oat flour
- One teaspoon of baking powder
- A pinch of salt

Instructions

1. Preheat the oven to 350° Fahrenheit.
2. Six muffin cups should be lined or greased with cooking oil.
3. Combine the olive oil, spinach, honey, eggs, and vanilla in a food processor. Blend until entirely smooth.
4. Whisk together the oat flour, almond flour, salt, baking soda, baking powder, and pepper in a medium mixing dish. Mix the spinach mixture well in the mixing cup.
5. Fill each muffin cup 2/3rd of the way with batter. Place the muffins in the oven for around 15 minutes or until gently browned and solid to the touch in the middle.
6. Remove the muffins from the pan and place them on a cooling rack to cool for 10 minutes before removing them.

7.16 Herb Scramble with Sautéed Cherry Tomatoes

Preparation time-5 minutes| Cook time-10 minutes| Total time-15 minutes| Servings-2|Difficulty-Easy

Nutritional Facts- Calories: 310; Total Fat: 26g; Total Carbohydrates: 10g; Sugar: 3g; Fiber: 5g; Protein: 13g; Sodium: 131mg

Ingredients

- Two teaspoons of chopped fresh oregano
- One cup of cherry tomatoes halved
- Half avocado, sliced
- Four eggs
- One tablespoon of extra-virgin olive oil
- Half garlic clove, sliced

Instructions

1. In a medium mixing cup, whisk together the eggs and oregano until well mixed.
2. Preheat a big skillet or pan to medium-high heat. Add the olive oil once the pan is warmed.
3. Pour the eggs into the pan and scramble them with a heat-resistant spatula or a wooden spoon. Place the eggs on a serving platter.
4. Cook for 2 minutes with the cherry tomatoes and garlic in the pan. Place the tomatoes on top of the eggs, then top with avocado slices.

7.17 Mushroom "Frittata"

Preparation time-15 minutes| Cook time-20 minutes| Total time-35 minutes| Servings-2|Difficulty-Easy

Nutritional Facts- Calories: 240; Total Fat: 8g; Total Carbohydrates: 34g; Sugar: 7g; Fiber: 10g; Protein: 11g; Sodium: 792mg

Ingredients

- Half cup of water

- One tablespoon of extra-virgin olive oil
- One pint of sliced mushrooms
- A pinch of ground cumin
- Half cup of chickpea flour
- A pinch of salt
- Half small red onion, diced
- A pinch of ground turmeric
- One tablespoon of chopped fresh parsley
- A pinch of freshly ground black pepper

Instructions

1. Preheat the oven to 350 degrees Fahrenheit.
2. Slowly whisk the water into the chickpea flour in a small bowl; season with salt and set aside.
3. Add the olive oil to big cast iron or oven-safe skillet or pan over high heat. Add the onion until the oil is heavy. Cook for 3 to 5 minutes, or until onion is softened and translucent. Add the mushrooms and cook for another 5 minutes. Sauté for 1 minute with the cumin, turmeric, pepper, and salt.
4. Sprinkle the parsley over the vegetables and pour the batter over them. Preheat the oven to 350°F and bake the skillet or pan for 20 to 25 minutes.
5. Serve hot.

7.18 Cucumber and Smoked-Salmon Lettuce Wraps

Preparation time-10 minutes| Cook time-0 minutes| Total time-10 minutes| Servings-2|Difficulty-Easy

Nutritional Facts- Calories: 107; Total Fat: 5g; Total Carbohydrates: 6g; Sugar: 4g; Fiber: 1g; Protein: 11g; Sodium: 1261mg

Ingredients

- Half English cucumber, sliced thin
- Four large butter lettuce leaves
- Four ounces of smoked salmon, divided
- Two tablespoons of Almost Caesar Salad Dressing, divided
- Half tablespoon of chopped fresh chives

Instructions

1. Arrange the lettuce leaves in a single sheet on a serving bowl.
2. Divide cucumber slices evenly throughout the lettuce leaves. 2 oz. smoked salmon on top of each leaf
3. Drizzle one tablespoon of Almost Caesar Salad Dressing over each wrap, and garnish with chives.

7.19 Sweet Potato Hash

Preparation time-15 minutes| Cook time-15 minutes| Total time-30 minutes| Servings-2|Difficulty-Easy

Nutritional Facts- Calories: 212; Total Fat: 7g; Total Carbohydrates: 35g; Sugar: 2g; Fiber: 6g; Protein: 30g; Sodium: 708mg

Ingredients

- Half onion, sliced thin
- One garlic clove, sliced thin
- Half cup of finely chopped Swiss chard
- A pinch of salt
- One tablespoon of coconut oil
- Half cup of sliced mushrooms
- One large sweet potato, cooked and cut into ½-inch cubes
- A quarter cup of vegetable broth
- A quarter teaspoon of freshly ground pepper
- Half tablespoon of chopped fresh sage
- Half tablespoon of chopped fresh thyme

Instructions

1. Melt the coconut oil in a big skillet or pan over a high flame.
2. Combine the mushrooms, onion, and garlic in a large mixing bowl. Cook, occasionally stirring, for around 8 minutes, or until the onions and mushrooms are soft.
3. Combine the Swiss chard, sweet potatoes, and vegetable broth in a large mixing bowl. Cook for around 5 minutes.
4. Add the salt, thyme, pepper, and sage, and mix well.

7.20 Fresh Berry Parfait with Coconut Cashew Cream

Preparation time-10 minutes| Cook time-0 minutes| Total time-10 minutes| Servings-2|Difficulty-Easy

Nutritional Facts- Calories: 200; Total Fat: 4g; Total Carbohydrates: 20g; Sugar: 2g; Fiber: 6g; Protein: 18g; Sodium: 308mg

Ingredients

- Half cup of unsweetened coconut milk
- One cup of raw cashews
- Two teaspoons of honey
- Two cups of berries (blackberries, blueberries, raspberries, strawberries)
- One teaspoon of ground cinnamon

Instructions

1. In a food processor, combine coconut milk, cashews, honey, and cinnamon. Blend until smooth, the consistency of which should be similar to fluffy peanut butter. If it's too dense, add a little water at a time and mix until it's the right consistency.
2. In the bottom of a shallow parfait glass, spoon two big spoonfuls of cashew cream.
3. Add half a cup of berries and another layer of cashew cream on top.
4. Add another half cup of berries to finish. In a second parfait glass, repeat the method.

7.21 Breakfast Burrito with Chickpeas and Avocado

Preparation time-15 minutes| Cook time-2 minutes| Total time-17 minutes| Servings-2|Difficulty-Easy

Nutritional Facts- Calories: 198; Total Fat: 6g; Total Carbohydrates: 26g; Sugar: 5g; Fiber: 9g; Protein: 22g; Sodium: 378mg

Ingredients

- One avocado
- One teaspoon of sea salt
- Half teaspoon of ground turmeric
- One (15-ounce) can of chickpeas, rinsed and drained
- One tablespoon of freshly squeezed lemon juice
- Half teaspoon of ground cumin
- Two tablespoons of sunflower seeds
- One cup of arugula, watercress, or microgreens
- Two brown rice or teff tortillas

Instructions

1. In a medium mixing bowl, put the chickpeas. Place the avocado in the bowl and mash it up. Combine the lemon juice, cumin, salt, and turmeric in a mixing bowl.
2. With a fork, mash the avocado into the mixture until it is fully incorporated. Allow a few entire chickpeas. Add the sunflower seeds and mix well.
3. Spray the tortillas with water and heat them in the microwave for 20 seconds just before eating. Half of the chickpea mixture should be placed in the middle of each tortilla. To make burritos, top the tortillas with arugula and roll them up like burritos.

7.22 Smoked Salmon and Avocado Tartine

Preparation time-10 minutes| Cook time-0 minutes| Total time-10 minutes| Servings-2|Difficulty-Easy

Nutritional Facts- Calories: 200; Total Fat: 4g; Total Carbohydrates: 20g; Sugar: 2g; Fiber: 6g; Protein: 18g; Sodium: 308mg

Ingredients

- Half tablespoon of freshly squeezed lime juice

- A pinch of sea salt
- Four ounces of smoked salmon or lox
- Two thinly sliced radishes
- Half avocado
- Half teaspoon of ground cumin
- Two slices of gluten-free bread, cut into quarters
- Half cup of alfalfa sprouts or microgreens

Instructions

1. In a medium bowl, mash the avocado. Mash in the cumin, lime juice, and salt with a fork until it is well mixed, but the mixture is always chunky.
2. Place two pieces of bread on each serving tray. On each slice, spread a layer of avocado mixture. Add half ounces of salmon on top.
3. Place some sprouts on top of the salmon and serve with radish slices as a garnish.

7.23 Breakfast Rice with Crumbled Nori

Preparation time-10 minutes| Cook time-0 minutes| Total time-10 minutes| Servings-2|Difficulty-Easy

Nutritional Facts- Calories: 200; Total Fat: 4g; Total Carbohydrates: 20g; Sugar: 2g; Fiber: 6g; Protein: 18g; Sodium: 308mg

Ingredients

- One teaspoon of coconut oil
- Half chopped shallot
- Half teaspoon of sea salt
- One cup of cooked brown rice
- One teaspoon of mirin
- One tablespoon of crumbled nori
- Half tablespoon of raw sesame seeds
- One crushed clove of garlic
- Three chopped cremini or button mushrooms
- Half cup of roughly chopped kale
- Half teaspoons of toasted sesame oil
- A quarter cup of chopped raw cashews

Instructions

1. Over medium heat, heat a large sauté pan. Toss in the sesame seeds and toast for 1 minute, or until lightly browned.

2. Cook, stirring regularly, until the oil, garlic, and shallot are soft and fragrant, for around 3 to 4 minutes.
3. Sauté the mushrooms with the salt until they are soft, around 3 minutes. Fold in the kale and stir until it begins to wilt around 3 to 4 minutes.
4. Stir in the sesame oil, rice, and mirin, and simmer for 2 minutes, or until the rice is cooked through. Cashews and nori are to be sprinkled on top.

7.24 Sweet Potato Hash with Lamb Sausage

Preparation time-10 minutes| Cook time-40 minutes| Total time-50 minutes| Servings-2|Difficulty-Moderate

Nutritional Facts- Calories: 200; Total Fat: 4g; Total Carbohydrates: 20g; Sugar: 2g; Fiber: 6g; Protein: 18g; Sodium: 308mg

Ingredients

- Half medium white or yellow onion, thinly sliced into half rings
- A quarter cup and two tablespoons of chopped cremini mushrooms
- One unpeeled garnet yam, cut into 1/4-inch cubes
- Two teaspoons of fresh thyme
- A pinch of ground sage
- A pinch of freshly ground black pepper
- One lamb sausages
- One teaspoon of sunflower oil (optional)
- One minced clove of garlic
- A quarter cup of finely chopped kale
- Half tablespoon of fresh oregano
- A pinch of sea salt

Instructions

1. Preheat oven to 375 degrees Fahrenheit.
2. In a big cast-iron skillet or pan over medium heat, squeeze the lamb out of its wrapping. Split the lamb into tiny parts with a spatula while it cooks and sauté until it browns around 4 minutes. You might need to apply some grapeseed or sunflower oil to the pan if you're using a leaner sausage, such as chicken. Move the sausage to a bowl using a slotted spoon.
3. Add the onion to the pan and cook for 4 to 5 minutes, or before it starts to caramelize. As required, drizzle in sunflower oil. Cook for three minutes, or until the mushrooms and garlic are softened.
4. Return the sausage to the skillet or pan with the yams, thyme, kale, oregano, salt, sage, and pepper.
5. Roast the yams in the skillet or pan in the oven for 20 to 25 minutes, or until quickly penetrated with a fork.

7.25 Sweet or Savory Quinoa Crepes

Preparation time-10 minutes| Cook time-10 minutes| Total time-20 minutes| Servings-2|Difficulty-Easy

Nutritional Facts- Calories: 200; Total Fat: 4g; Total Carbohydrates: 20g; Sugar: 2g; Fiber: 6g; Protein: 18g; Sodium: 308mg

Ingredients

- Two tablespoons of baking powder
- A quarter teaspoon of sea salt
- Two tablespoons of chia seeds
- One cup of unsweetened almond milk
- One teaspoon of freshly squeezed lemon juice
- Non-stick olive oil cooking spray
- Two cups of quinoa flour
- Half teaspoon of baking soda
- Half cup of raw cashews
- One and ¾ cups of water
- Two tablespoons of coconut oil
- One teaspoon of maple syrup

For sweet fillings

- Two and a half cups of stewed apples or pears with cinnamon
- Two and a half cups of mangoes blended with coconut milk
- Two and a half cups of fresh or frozen berries (thawed if frozen)
- Two cups of cashew cream (one and a half cups of raw cashews blended with Half a cup of water)

Savory fillings

- Two cups of hummus and one sliced avocado
- Two and a half cups of sautéed onions, mushrooms, and spinach
- Two ounces lox and One tablespoon of capers

Instructions

1. In a medium mixing cup, whisk together the flour, baking soda, baking powder, and salt. Grind the chia seeds and cashews until finely ground in a food processor or blender. Blend for 2 to 3 minutes with almond milk, water, lemon juice, oil, and maple syrup. Stir the wet ingredients into the dry ingredients until well combined. The quality of the batter should be similar to that of olive oil. If required, thin with more water.
2. Using oil, coat a medium non-stick plate, cast-iron skillet or pan, or crepe pan. Put around 2 to 3 teaspoons of crepe batter, swirled around in the pan until a thin crust forms around the

rim. Each crepe should be cooked for 1 minute on each hand. Cover with the filling of your choice.

7.26 Mango Muesli with Brazil Nut Topping

Preparation time-10 minutes| Refrigeration time-4 hours| Total time-4 hours and 10 minutes| Servings-2|Difficulty-Easy

Nutritional Facts- Calories: 386; Total Fat: 6g; Total Carbohydrates: 28g; Sugar: 7g; Fiber: 9g; Protein: 15g; Sodium: 374mg

Ingredients

- One cup of water
- Half cup of chopped mango
- A pinch of ground nutmeg
- A quarter cup of roughly chopped Brazil nuts
- ¾ cup of certified gluten-free oats
- Half cup of coconut milk, plus more for serving
- Half teaspoon of ground cinnamon
- A pinch of ground cardamom

Instructions

1. Combine the oats, coconut milk, cinnamon, nutmeg, mango, and cardamom in a big mixing bowl with a lid and stir well.
2. Refrigerate for at least 4 hours or overnight after covering. Serve with a dollop of coconut milk or cream and a handful of Brazil nuts on top.

7.27 Power-Packed Granola with Currants and Chia Seeds

Preparation time-10 minutes| Cook time-one hour| Total Time-One hour and 10 minutes| Servings-2|Difficulty-Hard

Nutritional Facts- Calories: 340; Total Fat: 8g; Total Carbohydrates: 25g; Sugar: 7g; Fiber: 5g; Protein: 30g; Sodium: 358mg

Ingredients

- One tablespoon of chia seeds
- Two tablespoons of agave nectar
- One and a quarter cup of certified gluten-free rolled oats
- Two tablespoons of coconut palm sugar
- One tablespoon of coconut oil
- A quarter cup of dried currants
- Half tablespoon of almond butter

Optional Additions

- A quarter cup of shelled pumpkin seeds (pepitas)
- A quarter cup of chopped pecans
- A quarter cup of unsweetened coconut flakes
- A quarter cup of dried cherries
- A quarter cup of raisins

Instructions

1. Preheat the oven to 300 ° F. and oil a baking sheet.
2. Combine the chia seeds, oats, agave, sugar, butter, and almond butter in a big mixing bowl and thoroughly combine. Pour the liquid into the tub and spread it out uniformly. Bake in the preheated oven for 40 minutes, stirring after 20 minutes.
3. Allow for the whole cooling before stirring in the currants and store in an airtight jar.

Chapter 8-Smoothie Recipes

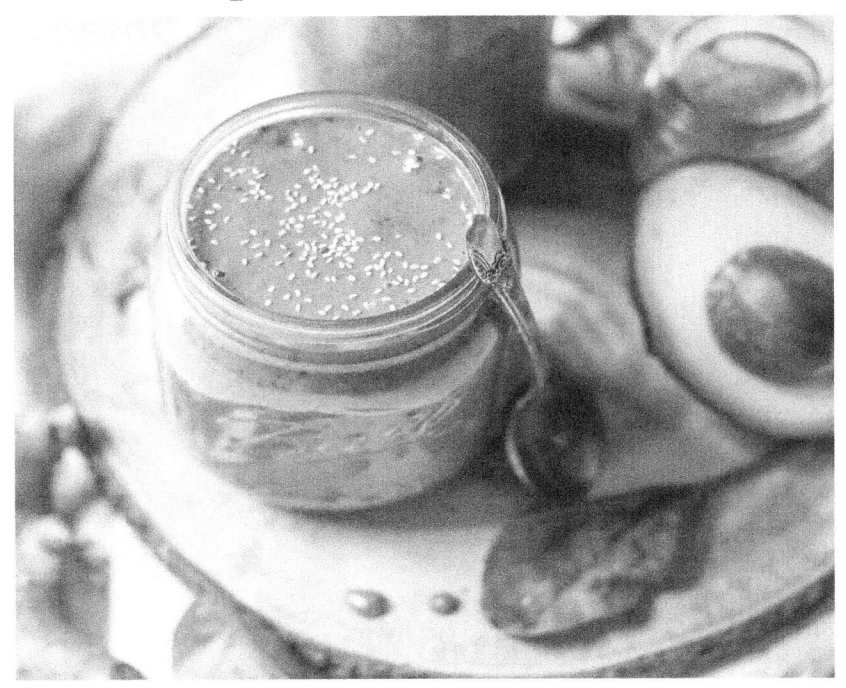

8.1 Inflammation-Soothing Smoothie

Preparation time-10 minutes| Cook time-0 minutes| Total time-10 minutes| Servings-2|Difficulty-Easy

Nutritional Facts- Calories: 147; Total Fat: 1g; Total Carbohydrates: 37g; Sugar: 6g; Fiber: 9g; Protein: 4g; Sodium: 89mg

Ingredients

- One fennel bulb
- Two cups of packed spinach
- Two cored and quartered pears
- Two thin slices of fresh ginger
- One cucumber, peeled if wax-coated or not organic
- Ice (optional)
- One cup of water

Instructions

1. In a blender, combine all the ingredients. Blend until smooth.
2. Serve the smoothie in two glasses and enjoy!

8.2 Kale and Banana Smoothie

Preparation time-5 minutes| Cook time-0 minutes| Total time-5 minutes| Servings-2|Difficulty-Easy

Nutritional Facts- Calories: 181; Total Fat: 4g; Total Carbs: 37g; Sugar: 15g; Fiber: 6g; Protein: 4g; Sodium: 210mg

Ingredients

- Two cups of stemmed and chopped kale
- Two packets of stevia
- One cup of crushed ice
- Two cups of unsweetened Almond milk
- Two peeled bananas
- One teaspoon of ground cinnamon

Instructions

1. In a blender, combine all the ingredients.
2. Blend until smooth.
3. Serve in two glasses and enjoy.

8.3 Eat-Your-Vegetables Smoothie

Preparation time-10 minutes| Cook time-0 minutes| Total time-10 minutes| Servings-2|Difficulty-Easy

Nutritional Facts- Calories: 140; Total Fat: 1g; Total Carbohydrates: 24g; Sugar: 23g; Fiber: 8g; Protein: 3g; Sodium: 293mg

Ingredients

- Two scrubbed and quartered small beets
- One cup of fresh raspberries
- Two trimmed carrot
- Two celery stalks
- Two cups of coconut water
- Ice (optional)
- Two teaspoons of balsamic vinegar

Instructions

1. In a blender, combine all the ingredients. Blend until smooth.
2. Blend until smooth.
3. Serve in two glasses and enjoy.

8.4 Cherry Smoothie

Preparation time-10 minutes| Cook time-0 minutes| Total time-10 minutes| Servings-2|Difficulty-Easy

Nutritional Facts- Calories: 266; Total Fat: 2g; Total Carbohydrates: 52g; Sugar: 48g; Fiber: 6g; Protein: 3g; Sodium: 122mg

Ingredients

- Half cup of fresh or frozen raspberries
- Two tablespoons of raw honey or maple syrup
- Two teaspoons of hemp seeds
- Ice (optional)
- Two cups of frozen no-added-sugar pitted cherries
- One and a quarter cup of coconut water
- Two teaspoons of chia seeds
- A drop of vanilla extract

Instructions

1. In a blender, combine all the ingredients.
2. Blend until smooth.
3. Serve in two glasses and enjoy.

8.5 Green Apple Smoothie

Preparation time-10 minutes| Cook time-0 minutes| Total time-10 minutes| Servings-2|Difficulty-Easy

Nutritional Facts- Calories: 176; Total Fat: 1g; Total Carbohydrates: 41g; Sugar: 34g; Fiber: 6g; Protein: 2g; Sodium: 110mg

Ingredients

- Two cored, seeded, and quartered green apples
- Half lemon, seeded
- One cup of coconut water
- Two cups of spinach
- One cucumber, peeled and seeded
- Ice (optional)
- Four teaspoons of raw honey or maple syrup

Instructions

1. In a blender, combine all the ingredients.
2. Blend until smooth.
3. Serve in two glasses and enjoy.

8.6 Turmeric and Green Tea Mango Smoothie

Preparation time-5 minutes| Cook time-0 minutes| Total time-5 minutes| Servings-2|Difficulty-Easy

Nutritional Facts- Calories: 285; Total Fat: 3g; Total Carbs: 68g; Sugar: 63g; Fiber: 6g; Protein: 4g; Sodium: 94mg

Ingredients

- Two teaspoons of turmeric powder
- Two cups of almond milk
- One cup of crushed ice
- Two cups of cubed mango
- Two tablespoons of matcha (green tea) powder
- Two tablespoons of honey

Instructions

1. In a blender, combine all the ingredients.
2. Blend until smooth.

8.7 Green Smoothie

Preparation time-5 minutes| Cook time-0 minutes| Total time-5 minutes|Servings-2|Difficulty-Easy

Nutritional Facts- Calories: 308; Total Fat: <1g; Total Carbs: 77g; Sugar: 61g; Fiber: 8g; Protein: 2g; Sodium: 50mg

Ingredients

- A quarter cup of cilantro leaves
- Three cups of unsweetened apple juice
- One cup of crushed ice
- Three cups of baby spinach
- Two peeled, cored, and chopped pears
- One tablespoon of grated ginger

Instructions

1. In a blender, combine all the ingredients.
2. Blend until smooth.
3. Serve in two glasses and enjoy.

8.8 One-for-All Smoothie

Preparation time-10 minutes| Cook time-0 minutes| Total time-10 minutes|Servings-2|Difficulty-Easy

Nutritional Facts- Calories: 152; Total Fat: 5g; Total Carbohydrates: 27g; Sugar: 15g; Fiber: 5g; Protein: 2g; Sodium: 90mg

Ingredients

- Half cup of fresh blueberries

- One cup of packed spinach
- Half banana
- Half teaspoon of vanilla extract
- One cup of coconut milk

Instructions

1. In a blender, combine all the ingredients.
2. Blend until smooth.

8.9 Mango-Thyme Smoothie

Preparation time-10 minutes| Cook time-0 minutes| Total time-10 minutes|Servings-2|Difficulty-Easy

Nutritional Facts- Calories: 274; Total Fat: 4g; Total Carbohydrates: 65g; Sugar: 54g; Fiber: 7g; Protein: 3g; Sodium: 125mg

Ingredients

- One cup of fresh seedless green grapes
- One cup of unsweetened almond milk
- Pinch sea salt
- Ice (optional)
- Two cups of fresh or frozen mango chunks
- Half fennel bulb
- One teaspoon of fresh thyme leaves
- Pinch freshly ground black pepper

Instructions

1. In a blender, combine all the ingredients.
2. Blend until smooth.
3. Serve in two glasses and enjoy.

8.10 Protein Powerhouse Smoothie

Preparation time-10 minutes| Cook time-0 minutes| Total time-10 minutes|Servings-2|Difficulty-Easy

Nutritional Facts- Calories: 500; Total Fat: 32g; Total Carbohydrates: 47g; Sugar: 34g; Fiber: 7g; Protein: 13g; Sodium: 199mg

Ingredients

- Two cups of fresh grapes
- Two tablespoons of hemp seed
- Half avocado

- Half cup of cashews (optional)
- Two to four mint leaves
- Ice (optional)
- Two cups of coconut milk

Instructions

1. In a blender, combine all the ingredients.
2. Blend until smooth.
3. Serve in two glasses and enjoy.

8.11 Chai Smoothie

Preparation time-10 minutes| Cook time-0 minutes| Total time-10 minutes|Servings-2|Difficulty-Easy

Nutritional Facts- Calories: 171; Total Fat: 4g; Total Carbohydrates: 35g; Sugar: 20g; Fiber: 5g; Protein: 3g; Sodium: 336mg

Ingredients

- Two pitted and chopped dates
- One teaspoon of the chai spice blend
- Two cups of unsweetened almond milk
- Half teaspoon of vanilla extract
- Pinch salt
- Ice cubes
- Two bananas, sliced into 1/4-inch rounds

Instructions

1. In a blender, combine all the ingredients.
2. Blend until smooth.
3. Serve in two glasses and enjoy.

8.12 Peachy Mint Punch

Preparation time-15 minutes| Cook time-0 minutes| Total time-15 minutes|Servings-2|Difficulty-Easy

Nutritional Facts- Calories: 81; Total Fat: 0g; Total Carbohydrates: 18g; Sugar: 14g; Fiber: 1g; Protein: 0g; Sodium: 85mg

Ingredients

- One and a half tablespoons of freshly squeezed lemon juice
- Half tablespoon of lemon zest
- One cup of sparkling water

- Ice
- Half of one (10-ounce) bag frozen no-added-sugar peach slices, thawed
- One and a half tablespoons of raw honey or maple syrup
- One cup of coconut water
- Two fresh mint sprigs, divided

Instructions

1. Combine the lemon juice, honey, peaches, and lemon zest in a food processor. Blend until entirely smooth.
2. Combine the coconut water and peach purée in a big pitcher. Place the mixture in the fridge to chill.
3. Fill two-wide (16-ounce) glasses of ice until ready to serve.
4. Add one sprig of mint to each bottle. Fill each glass with around a third of a cup of peach mixture and a splash of sparkling water.

8.13 Coconut-Ginger Smoothie

Preparation time-10 minutes| Cook time-0 minutes| Total time-10 minutes|Servings-2|Difficulty-Easy

Nutritional Facts-238; Total Fat: 18g; Total Carbohydrates: 16g; Sugar: 14g; Fiber: 10g; Protein: 5g; Sodium: 373mg

Ingredients

- One cup of coconut water
- Half cup of unsweetened coconut shreds or flakes
- Two thin slices of fresh ginger
- Ice (optional)
- One cup of coconut milk
- Half avocado
- Two teaspoons of raw honey or maple syrup
- Pinch ground cardamom (optional)

Instructions

1. In a blender, combine all the ingredients,
2. Blend until smooth.
3. Serve in two glasses and enjoy.

8.14 Super Green Smoothie

Preparation time-10 minutes| Cook time-0 minutes| Total time-10 minutes|Servings-2 |Difficulty-Easy

Nutritional Facts- Calories: 248; Total Fat: 14g; Total Carbohydrates: 33g; Sugar: 14g; Fiber: 10g; Protein: 5g; Sodium: 373mg

Ingredients

- One cucumber, peeled
- Half avocado
- Two cups of unsweetened almond milk
- Pinch salt
- Ice (optional)
- Two cups of packed spinach
- One pear
- Two teaspoons of raw honey or maple syrup
- Four mint leaves
- One lemon squeezed

Instructions

1. In a blender, combine all the ingredients.
2. Blend until smooth.
3. Serve in two glasses and enjoy.

8.15 Blueberry, Chocolate, and Turmeric Smoothie

Preparation time-5 minutes| Cook time-0 minutes| Total time-5 minutes|Servings-2|Difficulty-Easy

Nutritional Facts- Calories: 97; Total Fat: 5g; Total Carbs: 16g; Sugar: 7g; Fiber: 5g; Protein: 3g; Sodium: 182mg

Ingredients

- One cup of frozen wild blueberries
- One to two packets of stevia
- One cup of crushed ice
- Two cups of unsweetened almond milk
- Two tablespoons of cocoa powder
- One one-inch peeled piece of fresh turmeric

Instructions

1. In a blender, combine all the ingredients,
2. Blend until smooth.

8.16 Green Tea and Pear Smoothie

Preparation time-5 minutes| Cook time-0 minutes| Total time-5 minutes|Servings-2|Difficulty-Easy

Nutritional Facts- Calories: 208; Total Fat: 2g; Total Carbs: 51g; Sugar: 38g; Fiber: 7g; Protein: 1g; Sodium: 94mg

Ingredients

- Two peeled, cored, and chopped pears
- One one-inch piece of peeled and roughly chopped fresh ginger
- One cup of crushed ice
- Two cups of strongly brewed green tea
- Two tablespoons of honey
- One cup of unsweetened almond milk

Instructions

1. In a blender, combine all the ingredients.
2. Blend until smooth.

8.17 Ginger-Berry Smoothie

Preparation time-10 minutes| Cook time-0 minutes| Total time-10 minutes|Servings-2|Difficulty-Easy

Nutritional Facts- Calories: 95; Total Fat: 3g; Total Carbs: 16g; Sugar: 7g; Fiber: 9g; Protein: 3g; Sodium: 152mg

Ingredients

1. Two cups of unsweetened almond milk
2. Two cups of fresh blackberries
3. One to two packets of stevia
4. Two cups of crushed ice
5. One one-inch piece of peeled and roughly chopped ginger

Instructions

1. In a blender, combine all the ingredients.
2. Blend until smooth.

8.18 Berry Green Power Smoothie

Preparation time-5 minutes| Cook time-0 minutes| Total time-5 minutes|Servings-2|Difficulty-Easy

Nutritional Facts- Calories: 99; Total Fat: 2g; Total Carbs: 14g; Sugar: 8g; Fiber: 10g; Protein: 4g; Sodium: 166mg

Ingredients

- Two cups of frozen mixed berries
- Half cup of raw cashews
- Four tablespoons of chia seeds
- One cup of unsweetened hemp or almond milk
- Half teaspoon of minced fresh ginger
- Four cups of spinach or baby kale
- One banana
- Four mint leaves
- Half cup of water
- One teaspoon of honey

Instructions

1. In a blender, combine all the ingredients.
2. Blend until smooth.
3. Serve in two glasses and enjoy.

Chapter 9-Snacks and Appetizer Recipes

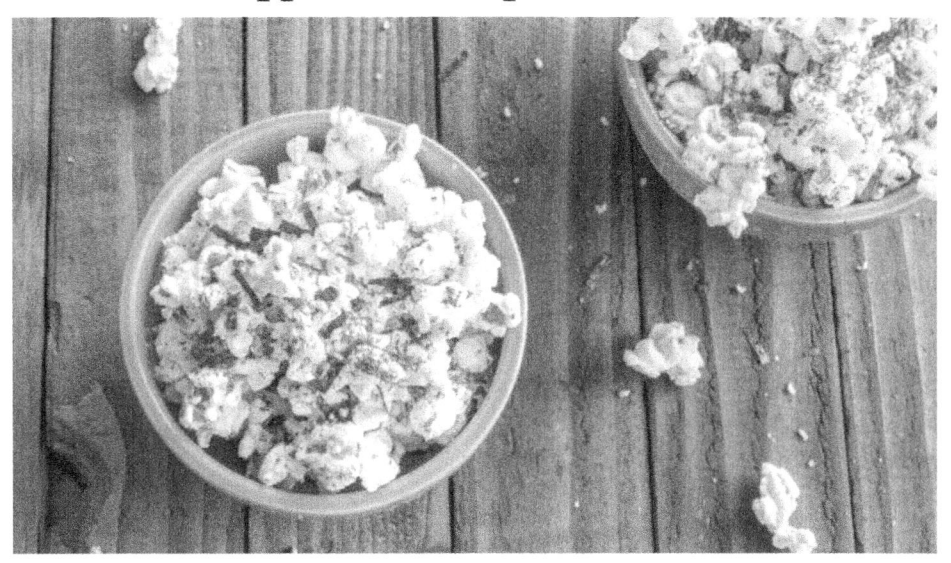

9.1 Cucumber-Yogurt Dip

Preparation time-15 minutes| Cook time-0 minutes| Total time-15 minutes| Servings-One cup |Difficulty-Easy

Nutritional Facts- Calories: 104; Total Fat: 9g; Total Carbohydrates: 7g; Sugar: 2g; Fiber: 3g; Protein: 1g; Sodium: 636mg

Ingredients

- One cup of plain coconut yogurt
- One chopped scallion
- One teaspoon of salt
- Two tablespoons of extra-virgin olive oil
- One peeled and shredded cucumber
- One minced garlic clove
- Two tablespoons of chopped fresh dill
- Two tablespoons of freshly squeezed lemon juice

Instructions

1. Drain the cucumber shredded in a fine-mesh strainer.
2. Combine the yogurt, garlic, salt, dill, scallion, and lemon juice in a shallow dish.
3. Fold in the cucumber that has been drained and serve in a serving dish.
4. Drizzle with olive oil only before serving.

9.2 White Bean Dip

Preparation time-15 minutes| Cook time-0 minutes| Total time-15 minutes| Servings-one cup| Difficulty-Easy

Nutritional Facts- Calories: 239; Total Fat: 14g; Total Carbohydrates: 25g; Sugar: 0g; Fiber: 6g; Protein: 9g; Sodium: 358mg

Ingredients

- One garlic clove
- Three tablespoons of extra-virgin olive oil
- One tablespoon of chopped fresh parsley
- Two tablespoons of freshly squeezed lemon juice
- One (15-ounce) can of white beans, drained and rinsed
- One tablespoon of tahini or almond butter
- A quarter cup of chopped pitted green olives
- A quarter teaspoon of salt

Instructions

1. Combine the garlic, white beans, and tahini in a food processor. Slowly drizzle in the olive oil in a small, continuous stream when the machine is on low. Thin the dip with a bit of water if it's too thick.
2. Combine the parsley, olives, and salt in a mixing bowl. To mix, pulse a few times. Add the lemon juice and mix well.
3. Serve with fresh veggies and gluten-free crackers in a serving dish.

9.3 Mashed Avocado with Jicama Slices

Preparation time-15 minutes| Cook time-0 minutes| Total time-15 minutes| Servings-2|Difficulty-Easy

Nutritional Facts- Calories: 270; Total Fat: 20g; Total Carbohydrates: 24g; Sugar: 4g; Fiber: 15g; Protein: 3g; Sodium: 595mg

Ingredients

- Half sliced scallion
- A pinch of ground turmeric
- Half teaspoon of salt
- Half jicama, peeled and cut into 1/4-inch-thick slices
- One pitted ripe avocado
- One tablespoon of chopped fresh cilantro
- Juice of half lemon
- Half teaspoon of freshly ground black pepper

Instructions

1. Combine the avocado, cilantro, scallion, turmeric, salt, lemon juice, and pepper in a small bowl. Mix the ingredients together, so they're well combined but always chunky.
2. Serve with jicama slices on the side.

9.4 Creamy Broccoli Dip

Preparation time-20 minutes| Cook time-5 minutes| Total time-25 minutes| Servings-One cup |Difficulty-Easy

Nutritional Facts- Calories: 82; Total Fat: 7g; Total Carbohydrates: 7g; Sugar: 1g; Fiber: 4g; Protein: 1g; Sodium: 628mg

Ingredients

- Half garlic clove
- Half cup of unsweetened almond yogurt or coconut yogurt
- Half tablespoon of freshly squeezed lemon juice
- Half cup of broccoli florets
- Half coarsely chopped scallion
- A quarter avocado
- Half teaspoon of salt
- Pinch red pepper flakes
- Half teaspoon of dried dill

Instructions

1. Fill a medium pot halfway with water, set it over medium-high heat, and put a steamer basket inside.
2. Fill the steamer basket halfway with broccoli, cover, and steam for 5 minutes, or until the broccoli is bright green. Drain the broccoli and remove the pan from the heat.
3. Combine the garlic, yogurt, scallion, avocado, dill, salt, lemon juice, and red pepper flakes in a food processor. Pulse the paste a couple of times, so it seems coarsely sliced.
4. Process before the broccoli is well combined; the mixture can retain some structure and not be totally puréed.
5. Serve with Sweet Potato Chips or carrot and celery sticks as a side dish.

9.5 Smoked Trout and Mango Wraps

Preparation time-15 minutes| Cook time-0 minutes| Total time-15 minutes| Servings-2|Difficulty-Easy

Nutritional Facts- Calories: 108; Total Fat: 3g; Total Carbohydrates: 13g; Sugar: 10g; Fiber: 3g; Protein: 9g; Sodium: 52mg

Ingredients

- Two ounces smoked trout, divided
- Two large green-leaf lettuce leaves, thick stems removed
- Half cup of chopped mango, divided
- One tablespoon of freshly squeezed lemon juice, divided
- Half sliced scallion

Instructions

1. On a flat surface, arrange the lettuce leaves. Bits of trout and mango are to be evenly distributed on each leaf. Scallions should be sprinkled on top, and lemon juice should be drizzled on top.
2. Burrito-style wrap the lettuce leaves and arrange them seam-side down on a serving tray.

9.6 Kale Chips

Preparation time-20minutes|Cook time-20 minutes| Total time-40 minutes|Servings-2|Difficulty-Moderate

Nutritional Facts- Calories: 93; Total Fat: 7g; Total Carbohydrates: 7g; Sugar: 0g; Fiber: 1g; Protein: 2g; Sodium: 497mg

Ingredients

- One tablespoon of extra-virgin olive oil
- Half bunch kale, thoroughly washed and dried, ribs removed, and cut into 2-inch strips
- Half teaspoon of sea salt

Instructions

1. Preheat the oven to 275 degrees Fahrenheit.
2. Mix the olive oil and kale in a big mixing bowl using your hands until the kale is finely covered with the oil.
3. Place the kale on a baking sheet and spread it out in a single layer. Season with a pinch of salt.
4. Bake for around 20 minutes, or until the kale is crisp, on a preheated baking dish. Halfway through the baking time, flip the chips over to crisp the other hand.
5. Until eating, enable the chips to cool slightly.

9.7 Smoked Turkey–Wrapped Zucchini Sticks

Preparation time-10 minutes| Cook time-0 minutes| Total time-10 minutes| Servings-2|Difficulty-Easy

Nutritional Facts- Calories: 137; Total Fat: 3g; Total Carbohydrates: 6g; Sugar: 2g; Fiber: 1g; Protein: 21g; Sodium: 1450mg

Ingredients

- One quartered lengthwise zucchini
- Pinch salt
- Four thin slices of smoked turkey
- Half cup of packed arugula, divided

Instructions

1. Place one smoked turkey slice on a work surface. Add one zucchini stick, a quarter cup of arugula, and a pinch of salt to the top.
2. Wrap the turkey around the veggies and put seam-side down on a platter. Repeat for the rest of the ingredients.

3. Refrigerate before ready to eat.

9.8 Crunchy-Spicy Chickpeas

Preparation time-10 minutes| Cook time-40 minutes| Total time-50 minutes| Servings-One cup| Difficulty-Moderate

Nutritional Facts- Calories: 192; Total Fat: 10g; Total Carbohydrates: 18g; Sugar: 1g; Fiber: 5g; Protein: 8g; Sodium: 593mg

Ingredients

- One teaspoon of salt
- Half teaspoon of onion powder
- Half teaspoon of chipotle powder
- Two tablespoons of extra-virgin olive oil
- One (15-ounce) can chickpeas, drained
- Half teaspoon of ground cumin
- Half teaspoon of ground turmeric
- A quarter teaspoon of garlic powder

Instructions

1. Preheat the oven to 375 degrees Fahrenheit.
2. Using a paper towel, pat dry the drained chickpeas.
3. Combine the salt, onion powder, cumin, chipotle powder, turmeric, and garlic powder in a shallow cup.
4. Combine the dried chickpeas and olive oil in a medium mixing dish. Gently toss the chickpeas in the oil to cover them.
5. Over the chickpeas, sprinkle the salt mixture. Stir until it is uniformly coated.
6. Spread the chickpeas in a single layer on a wide baking sheet with elevated sides (to prevent the chickpeas from falling off the sheet). Place the sheet in the preheated oven and bake for 30 to 40 minutes, or until the chickpeas are dry and crunchy, stirring periodically.
7. Until feeding, allow cooling fully.

9.9 Sweet Potato Chips

Preparation time-20 minutes| Cook time-2 hours| Total time-2 hours and 20 minutes| Servings-2|Difficulty-Hard

Nutritional Facts- Calories: 267; Total Fat: 11g; Total Carbohydrates: 42g; Sugar: 1g; Fiber: 6g; Protein: 2g; Sodium: 482mg

Ingredients

- One large sweet potato, sliced as thin as possible
- Half teaspoon of sea salt
- One and a half tablespoons of extra-virgin olive oil

Instructions

1. Preheat the oven to 250 degrees Fahrenheit.
2. Place the oven rack in the middle of the oven.
3. Toss the sweet potato slices with olive oil in a big mixing bowl. Arrange the slices on two baking sheets in a single layer. Season with a pinch of salt.
4. Bake the sheets for around 2 hours in a preheated oven, turning the pans and tossing the chips after an hour.
5. Pull the chips from the oven until they are finely browned and crisp. Some might be a little fluffy at first, but when they cool, they can crisp up. Allow 10 minutes for the chips to cool before serving.
6. Serve right away. Within a few hours, the chips have lost their crunch.

9.10 Mini Snack Muffins

Preparation time-20 minutes| Cook time-20 minutes| Total time-40 minutes| Servings-6 muffins |Difficulty-Easy

Nutritional Facts- Calories: 65; Total Fat: 4g; Total Carbohydrates: 7g; Sugar: 1g; Fiber: 1g; Protein: 2g; Sodium: 66mg

Ingredients

- A quarter cup of almond flour
- A quarter tablespoon of baking powder
- A quarter teaspoon of ground cinnamon
- A quarter cup of extra-virgin olive oil, plus extra for greasing
- A quarter cup of brown rice flour
- A pinch teaspoon of salt
- One egg
- A quarter cup of canned pumpkin
- A quarter cup of shredded carrot

Instructions

1. Preheat the oven to 375 degrees Fahrenheit.
2. Using cupcake liners or a little olive oil, fill a mini-muffin tin with cupcake liners.
3. Combine the almond flour, salt, baking powder, brown rice flour, and cinnamon in a medium mixing bowl.
4. Combine the eggs, pumpkin, carrots, and olive oil in a mixing bowl. Stir before it is well blended.
5. Scoop about three-quarters of the batter into each muffin cup.
6. Bake the muffins for 15 minutes, or until lightly browned. Remove the muffins from the tin and let them cool for 10 minutes before removing them from the oven.

9.11 Strawberry-Chia Ice Pops

Preparation time-20 minutes| Freeze time-5 hours| Total time-15 minutes| Servings-2 ice pops| Difficulty-Easy

Nutritional Facts- Calories: 187; Total Fat: 17g; Total Carbohydrates: 9g; Sugar: 6g; Fiber: 3g; Protein: 2g; Sodium: 11mg

Ingredients

- Half tablespoon of freshly squeezed lemon juice
- One cup of frozen unsweetened strawberries, thawed
- Half of one (15-ounce) can of coconut milk
- Half teaspoon of vanilla extract
- Half tablespoon of chia seeds

Instructions

1. Follow the manufacturer's guidance to make two ice pop molds.
2. Combine the strawberries, chia seeds, coconut milk, lemon juice, and vanilla in a medium mixing cup. Allow the mixture to sit for 5 minutes to thicken slightly due to the chia seeds. This makes filling the molds a lot smoother.
3. Distribute the mixture evenly among the molds. In each mold, place one ice pop stick. Freeze the pops for 5 hours or overnight until they are strong.

9.12 Garlic Ranch Dip

Preparation time-15 minutes| Cook time-0 minutes| Total time-15 minutes| Servings-One cup |Difficulty-Easy

Nutritional Facts- Calories: 69; Total Fat: 5g; Total Carbs: 6g; Sugar: 2g; Fiber: <1g; Protein: 1g; Sodium:357mg

Ingredients

- A quarter cup of buttermilk
- One tablespoon of chopped fresh chives
- A quarter cup of anti-inflammatory mayonnaise
- Three minced garlic cloves
- One tablespoon of chopped fresh dill
- A quarter teaspoon of freshly ground black pepper
- Half teaspoon of sea salt

Instructions

1. In a small bowl, stir together all the ingredients.

9.13 Blueberry Nut Trail Mix

Preparation time-5 minutes| Cook time-5 minutes| Total time-10 minutes| Servings-2|Difficulty-Easy

Nutritional Facts- Calories: 179; Total Fat: 16g; Total Carbs: 8g; Sugar: 3g; Fiber: 3g; Protein: 5g; Sodium: 39mg

Ingredients

- Half cup of almonds
- Half tablespoon of extra-virgin olive oil
- Pinch salt
- A quarter cup of dried blueberries
- A quarter teaspoon of Chinese Five-spice powder

Instructions

1. Heat the olive oil in a big nonstick skillet or pan over medium-high heat until it starts shimmering.
2. Cook for 2 minutes, stirring regularly, after adding the salt, almonds, and Chinese five-spice.
3. Remove from the heat and set aside to cool. Add the blueberries and stir to combine.

9.14 Black Bean and Artichoke Hummus

Preparation time-15 minutes| Cook time-0 minutes| Total time-15 minutes| Servings-2|Difficulty-Easy

Nutritional Facts- Calories: 199; Total Fat: 18g; Total Carbs: 9g; Sugar: 4g; Fiber: 4g; Protein: 7g; Sodium: 40mg

Ingredients

- Half of one (6-ounce) jar artichoke hearts marinated in olive oil
- Half tablespoon of tahini
- Half teaspoon of sea salt
- Half of one (15-ounce) can of black beans, rinsed and drained
- One minced garlic clove
- One and a half tablespoons of extra-virgin olive oil

Instructions

1. In a food processor, combine the beans, garlic, oil, artichokes, and tahini. Slowly drizzle in the oil when the engine is working and mix to the perfect quality. Season with salt.
2. Serve with zucchini, carrots, cucumbers, jicama, snap peas or daikon radishes as a side dish.

9.15 Crispy Curried Chickpeas

Preparation time-15 minutes| Cook time-40 minutes| Total time-55 minutes| Servings-2|Difficulty-Moderate

Nutritional Facts- Calories: 192; Total Fat: 10g; Total Carbohydrates: 18g; Sugar: 1g; Fiber: 5g; Protein: 8g; Sodium: 593mg

Ingredients

- Half tablespoon of grapeseed oil

- Half teaspoon of ground turmeric
- Half of one (15-ounce) can chickpeas, rinsed and drained
- One teaspoon of ground cumin
- Half teaspoon of sea salt
- A quarter teaspoon of fenugreek
- A quarter teaspoon of freshly ground black pepper

Instructions

1. Preheat oven to 400 degrees Fahrenheit.
2. Place the chickpeas in a medium bowl after patting them dry with a paper towel. Whisk together the oil, turmeric, cumin, pepper, salt, and fenugreek in a wide bowl with a fork. Stir the chickpeas in the oil mixture until they are well seasoned.
3. Bake the chickpeas in a baking pan for 40 minutes, or until golden brown and rattling around the pan.
4. Serve right away, or allow to cool completely before storage in an airtight jar.

9.16 White Bean and Kalamata Olive Hummus

Preparation time-15 minutes| Cook time-0 minutes| Total time-15 minutes| Servings-2|Difficulty-Easy

Nutritional Facts- Calories: 210; Total Fat: 12g; Total Carbohydrates: 20g; Sugar: 1g; Fiber: 6g; Protein: 8g; Sodium: 563mg

Ingredients

- One clove of garlic
- One and a half tablespoons of extra-virgin olive oil
- Half teaspoon of sea salt
- Half of one (15-ounce can) cannellini or other white beans, rinsed and drained
- Half tablespoon of tahini
- A quarter cup of pitted kalamata olives

Instructions

1. In a food processor, combine the garlic, beans, and tahini. Slowly drizzle in the oil when the engine is working and mix to the perfect quality. Pulse in the olives before they are finely sliced and added. Season with salt and pepper.
2. Serve with carrots, cucumbers, jicama, snap peas, zucchini, or daikon radishes as a side dish.

9.17 Shiitake Mushroom and Walnut Pâté

Preparation time-10 minutes| Cook time-17 minutes| Total time-27 minutes| Servings-2|Difficulty-Easy

Nutritional Facts- Calories: 192; Total Fat: 10g; Total Carbohydrates: 18g; Sugar: 1g; Fiber: 5g; Protein: 8g; Sodium: 593mg

Ingredients

- Half tablespoon of coconut oil
- A quarter teaspoon of sea salt, divided
- Half teaspoon of maple syrup
- Half cup of raw walnuts
- Two sliced shiitake mushrooms
- A quarter cup of cooked butter beans or other white beans

Instructions

1. Preheat oven to 350 degrees Fahrenheit.
2. Spread the walnuts out on a baking sheet and bake for 12 minutes or until they begin to brown and smell nice. Afterward, remove and set it aside.
3. Heat the oil in a shallow sauté pan. Cook, stirring regularly, for around 5 minutes, until the mushrooms are tender and juicy, seasoning with a quarter teaspoon of salt.
4. In a food processor, puree the walnuts, beans, mushrooms, maple syrup, and the remaining salt until creamy. The finished product would be thick and similar to liver pâté.
5. Serve with rice crackers or mixed veggies.

9.18 Creamy Avocado Spinach Dip

Preparation time-15 minutes| Cook time-0 minutes| Total time-15 minutes| Servings-One cup| Difficulty-Easy

Nutritional Facts- Calories: 188; Total Fat: 13g; Total Carbohydrates: 21g; Sugar: 2g; Fiber: 6g; Protein: 9g; Sodium: 433mg

Ingredients

- One cup of spinach
- A quarter cup of olive oil, plus more as needed
- Half teaspoon of ground cumin
- A quarter cup of pitted kalamata olives (optional)
- Half avocado
- One chopped clove of garlic
- One tablespoon of freshly squeezed lemon
- Half teaspoon of sea salt

Instructions

1. Fill a food processor halfway with avocado. Blend in the garlic, spinach, and oil. If you want a more refined finish, apply more oil. Blend in the cumin, lemon juice, and salt until almost smooth. Pulse in the olives before they are finely sliced and integrated.

2. Assorted vegetables, such as cucumbers, carrots, cauliflower, or jicama, may be served alongside. This dip is often delicious as a sandwich spread or as a garnish for bean and rice dishes.

9.19 Artichoke and Basil Tapenade

Preparation time-15 minutes| Cook time-0 minutes| Total time-15 minutes| Servings-2|Difficulty-Easy

Nutritional Facts- Calories: 179; Total Fat: 7g; Total Carbohydrates: 15g; Sugar: 2g; Fiber: 12g; Protein: 9g; Sodium: 472mg

Ingredients

- A quarter cup of pitted green olives
- Two to four large basil leaves
- Half of one (14-ounce) jar artichoke hearts marinated in olive oil
- A quarter cup of pitted kalamata olives

Instructions

1. In a blender or food processor, pulse all of the ingredients until finely minced but not pureed.
2. Assorted vegetables, such as cauliflower, carrots, or celery, can be served alongside.

9.20 Anti-Inflammatory Trail Mix

Preparation time-15 minutes| Cook time-0 minutes| Total time-15 minutes| Servings-2 snack pouches |Difficulty-Easy

Nutritional Facts- Calories: 210; Total Fat: 9g; Total Carbohydrates: 20g; Sugar: 2g; Fiber: 15g; Protein: 9g; Sodium: 528mg

Ingredients

- Two tablespoons of shelled pistachios
- Two tablespoons of raw almonds
- One tablespoon of shelled pumpkin seeds (pepitas)
- One tablespoon of chopped unsweetened, unsulfured dried mangoes
- One tablespoon of freeze-dried blueberries

Optional additions

- Two tablespoons of pecans
- Two tablespoons of Brazil nuts
- Two tablespoons of sunflower seeds
- One tablespoon of raisins
- One tablespoon of dried apricots
- Two tablespoons of freeze-dried raspberries
- Two tablespoons of walnuts

- Two tablespoons of macadamia nuts
- Two tablespoons of unsweetened coconut flakes
- One tablespoon of dried figs
- Two tablespoons of freeze-dried strawberries

Instructions

1. Toss the almonds, pumpkin seeds pistachios, pistachios, blueberries, and mangoes together in a big mixing bowl. Put some optional ingredients in small bowls and place them on the table for people to pick from.
2. In a quarter-cup measuring cup, combine a little of each desired ingredient and dump the contents into snack bags for pre-portioned, power-packed snacks that are ready to catch and go!

9.21 Nutty Coconut Energy Truffle

Preparation time-15 minutes| Cook time-0 minutes| Total time-15 minutes| Servings-2 |Difficulty-Easy

Nutritional Facts- Calories: 212; Total Fat: 10g; Total Carbohydrates: 21g; Sugar: 3g; Fiber: 17g; Protein: 11g; Sodium: 456mg

Ingredients

- One and a half teaspoon of ground cinnamon
- Two tablespoons of pitted dates
- Half tablespoon of coconut oil
- 1/8 teaspoon of almond extract
- Two tablespoons of unsweetened shredded coconut
- Half cup of raw walnuts
- 1/8 teaspoon of sea salt
- Two tablespoons of dried cherries
- Half tablespoon of almond butter
- Half tablespoon of maple syrup (optional)

Instructions

1. In a food processor, combine the cinnamon, walnuts, and salt. Process for 1 minute, or until the nuts are finely ground.
2. Combine the cherries, dates, almond butter, oil, and extract in a mixing bowl. Process before it is well combined; the mixture should be dense and sticky. Fold any of the mixtures in your hands and see how it can be shaped into a truffle; if it falls apart quickly, add the maple syrup.
3. Place the coconut on a plate and spread it out. Using a big spoon, scoop the nut mixture and roll it into 1-inch cubes. Roll the balls in the coconut until they are fully covered.
4. In case you make more than two servings, you can refrigerate the truffles for up to one week in an airtight bag and freeze any leftovers for up to six months.

9.22 Tropical Quinoa Power Bars

Preparation time-10 minutes| Cook time-20 minutes| Total time-30 minutes| Servings-2 |Difficulty-Easy

Nutritional Facts- Calories: 201; Total Fat: 13g; Total Carbohydrates: 23g; Sugar: 3g; Fiber: 11g; Protein: 16g; Sodium: 556mg

Ingredients

- A quarter cup of quinoa, rinsed and drained
- Two tablespoons of raw macadamia nuts
- Two tablespoons of chopped dried apricots
- Half tablespoon of tahini
- One tablespoon of coconut flour
- Half cups of water
- A pinch of sea salt
- Two tablespoons of unsweetened shredded coconut
- Half tablespoon of honey
- Half teaspoon of ground cinnamon

Instructions

1. In a medium saucepan over medium-high heat, combine the quinoa, water, and salt. Bring to a boil, then reduce to a low heat environment. Cook for 20 minutes, stirring occasionally. The quinoa would seem to have sprouted and grown a tiny tail, and all of the liquid may have been drained. Enable to cool for around 5 minutes after fluffing with a fork.
2. Combine quinoa, coconut, macadamia nuts, and apricots in a big mixing bowl. Combine the tahini, honey, and cinnamon in a mixing bowl. Cover with the coconut flour and knead it together with your hands until all is well combined.
3. Shape the mixture into bars that are around 3 inches long and 1 inch wide. Cover and refrigerate for 4 hours or overnight in a shallow baking pan lined with parchment paper.

Chapter 10-Lunch Recipes

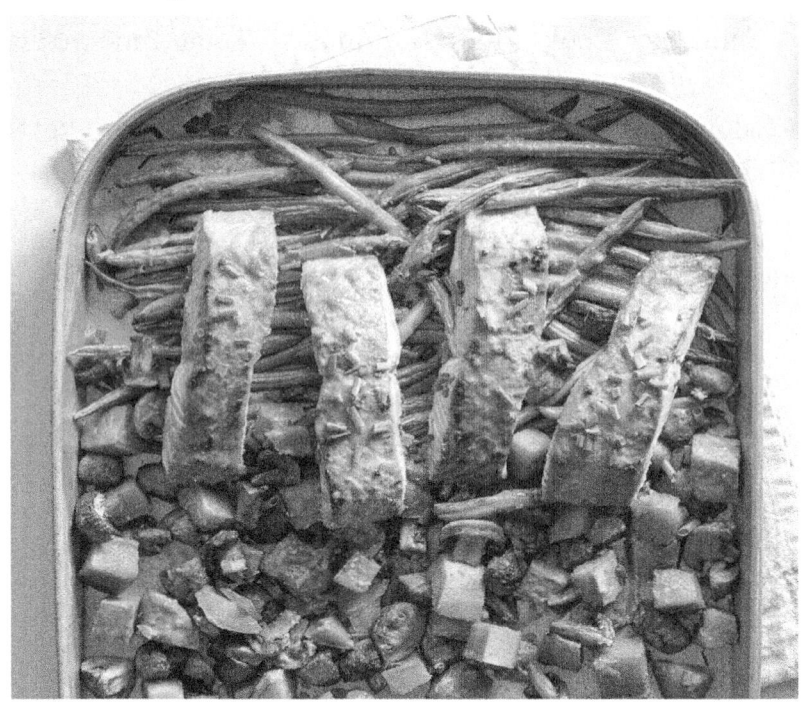

10.1 Lentils with Tomatoes and Turmeric

Preparation time-10 minutes| Cook time-10 minutes| Total time-20 minutes| Servings-2|Difficulty-Easy

Nutritional Facts- Calories: 248; Total Fat: 8g; Total Carbs: 34g; Sugar: 5g; Fiber: 15g; Protein: 12g; Sodium 243mg

Ingredients

- Half finely chopped onion
- Half teaspoon of garlic powder
- Half of one (14-ounce) can of chopped tomatoes, drained
- 1/8 teaspoon of freshly ground black pepper
- One tablespoon of extra-virgin olive oil, plus extra for garnish
- Half tablespoon of ground turmeric
- Half of one (14-ounce) can of lentils, drained
- A quarter teaspoon of sea salt

Instructions

1. Heat the olive oil in a big pot over medium-high heat until it starts shimmering.
2. Cook, stirring regularly, for around 5 minutes, or until the onion and turmeric are tender.
3. Add the garlic powder, salt, tomatoes, lentils, and pepper.
4. Cook, stirring regularly, for 5 minutes. If required, serve with a drizzle of extra virgin olive oil on top.

10.2 Fried Rice with Kale

Preparation time-10 minutes| Cook time-12 minutes| Total time-22 minutes| Servings-2|Difficulty-Easy

Nutritional Facts- Calories: 301; Total Fat: 11g; Total Carbs: 36g; Sugar: 1g; Fiber: 3g; Protein: 16g; Sodium: 2,535mg

Ingredients

- Four ounces of chopped tofu
- One cup of stemmed and chopped Kale
- Two tablespoons of stir-fry sauce
- One tablespoon of extra-virgin olive oil
- Three sliced scallions
- One and a half cups of cooked brown rice

Instructions

1. Heat the olive oil in a big skillet or pan over medium-high heat until it starts shimmering.
2. Add the scallions, tofu, and kale. Cook, stirring regularly, for 5 to 7 minutes, or until the vegetables are tender.
3. Combine the stir-fry sauce and brown rice in a mixing bowl. Cook, stirring regularly, for 3 to 5 minutes, or until thoroughly heated.

10.3 Tofu and Red Pepper Stir-Fry

Preparation time-10 minutes| Cook time-11 minutes| Total time-21 minutes| Servings-2|Difficulty-Easy

Nutritional Facts- Calories: 166; Total Fat: 10g; Total Carbs: 17g; Sugar: 12g; Fiber: 2g; Protein: 7g; Sodium: 892mg

Ingredients

- One chopped red bell peppers
- One tablespoon of extra-virgin olive oil
- Half chopped onion
- A quarter cup of ginger teriyaki sauce
- Four ounces of chopped tofu

Instructions

1. Heat the olive oil in a big skillet or pan over medium-high heat until it starts shimmering.
2. Add the onion, red bell peppers, and tofu. Cook, stirring regularly, for 5 to 7 minutes, or until the vegetables are soft and beginning to brown.
3. Apply the teriyaki sauce to the skillet or pan after whisking it together. Cook, sometimes stirring, for 3 to 4 minutes, or until the sauce thickens.

10.4 Sweet Potato and Bell Pepper Hash with a Fried Egg

Preparation time-5 minutes| Cook time-25 minutes| Total time-30 minutes| Servings-2|Difficulty-Easy

Nutritional Facts- Calories: 384; Total Fat: 19g; Total Carbs: 47g; Sugar: 16g; Fiber: 8g; Protein: 10g; Sodium: 603mg

Ingredients

- Half chopped onion
- Two cups of peeled and cubed potatoes
- Two tablespoons of extra-virgin olive oil
- Half chopped red bell pepper
- Half teaspoon of sea salt
- Two eggs
- A pinch of freshly ground black pepper

Instructions

1. Heat one tablespoon of olive oil in a big non-stick pan over medium-high heat until it starts shimmering.
2. Add the red bell pepper, onion, and sweet potato. Season with salt and a pinch of black pepper. Cook, stirring regularly, for 15 to 20 minutes, or until the potatoes are soft and browned. Serve the potatoes in four bowls.
3. Return the skillet or pan to heat, turn the heat down to medium-low, and swirl to cover the bottom of the pan with the remaining one tablespoon of olive oil.
4. Scatter some salt over the eggs and carefully smash them into the tray. Cook until the whites are set, around 3 to 4 minutes. Flip the eggs gently and remove them from the heat. Allow 1 minute for the eggs to rest in the hot skillet or pan. One egg should be placed on top of each serving of hash.

10.5 Quinoa Florentine

Preparation time-5 minutes| Cook time-25 minutes| Total time-30 minutes| Servings-2|Difficulty-Easy

Nutritional Facts- Calories: 403; Total Fat: 12g; Total Carbs: 62g; Sugar: 4g; Fiber: 7g; Protein: 13g; Sodium: 278mg

Ingredients

- Half chopped onion
- Two minced garlic cloves
- Two cups of no-salt-added vegetable broth
- A pinch of freshly ground black pepper
- One tablespoon of extra-virgin olive oil
- One and a half cups of fresh baby spinach

- One cup of quinoa rinsed well
- A quarter teaspoon of sea salt

Instructions

1. Heat the olive oil in a big pot over medium-high heat until it starts shimmering.
2. Add the spinach and onion. Cook, stirring regularly, for 3 minutes.
3. Cook, stirring continuously, for 30 seconds after adding the garlic.
4. Combine the vegetable broth, salt, quinoa, and pepper in a mixing bowl. Bring to a simmer, then reduce to low heat. Cook, covered, for 15 to 20 minutes, or until the liquid has been absorbed. Using a fork, fluff the mixture.

10.6 Tomato Asparagus Frittata

Preparation time-10 minutes| Cook time-10 minutes| Total time-20 minutes| Servings-2|Difficulty-Easy

Nutritional Facts-Calories: 224; Total Fat: 14g; Total Carbs: 15g; Sugar: 10g; Fiber: 5g; Protein: 12g; Sodium: 343mg

Ingredients

- Five trimmed asparagus spears
- Three eggs
- One tablespoon of extra-virgin olive oil
- Five Cherry Tomatoes
- Half tablespoon of chopped fresh thyme
- A pinch of freshly ground black pepper
- A quarter teaspoon of sea salt

Instructions

1. Preheat the broiler to the highest setting.
2. Heat the olive oil in a big ovenproof skillet or pan over medium-high heat until it starts shimmering.
3. Toss in the asparagus. Cook, stirring regularly, for 5 minutes.
4. Toss in the tomatoes. Cook for 3 minutes, stirring once in a while.
5. Whisk together the thyme, salt, eggs, and pepper in a medium mixing cup. Carefully spill over the tomatoes and asparagus, turning them about in the pan to ensure that they are equally distributed.
6. Turn the heat down to medium. Cook for 3 minutes, or until the eggs are hardened around the outside. Carefully draw the eggs away from the skillet or pan's sides with a rubber spatula, then tilt the pan to allow the uncooked eggs to run into the edges. Cook for 3 minutes, or until the edges are set.
7. Place the pan under the broiler and cook for 3 to 5 minutes, or until puffed and brown. To eat, cut into wedges.

10.7 Tofu Sloppy Joes

Preparation time-10 minutes| Cook time-15 minutes| Total time-25 minutes| Servings-2|Difficulty-Easy

Nutritional Facts- Calories: 209; Total Fat: 10g; Total Carbs: 21g; Sugar: 13g; Fiber: 8g; Protein: 11g; Sodium: 644mg

Ingredients

- Half chopped onion
- One (14-ounce) can of crushed Tomatoes
- Half tablespoon of chili powder
- One tablespoon of extra-virgin olive oil
- Five ounces of chopped Tofu
- Two tablespoons of apple cider vinegar
- Half teaspoon of garlic powder
- A pinch of freshly ground black pepper
- A quarter teaspoon of sea salt

Instructions

1. Heat the olive oil in a big pot over medium-high heat until it starts shimmering.
2. Combine the tofu and onion in a mixing bowl. Cook, stirring regularly, for around 5 minutes, or until the onion is tender.
3. Combine the tomatoes, apple cider vinegar, salt, garlic powder, chili powder, and pepper in a large mixing bowl. Simmer for 10 minutes, stirring regularly, to enable the flavors to meld.

10.8 Broccoli and Egg "Muffins"

Preparation time-10 minutes| Cook time-20 minutes| Total time-30 minutes| Servings-2|Difficulty-Easy

Nutritional Facts- Calories: 207; Total Fat: 16; Total Carbs: 5g; Sugar: 2g; Fiber: 1g; Protein: 12g; Sodium: 366mg

Ingredients

- One tablespoon of extra-virgin olive oil
- Half cup of chopped broccoli florets
- Half teaspoon of garlic powder
- Two tablespoons of freshly ground black pepper
- Non-stick cooking spray
- Half chopped onion
- Four beaten eggs
- A quarter teaspoon of sea salt

Instructions

1. Preheat the oven to 350 degrees Fahrenheit.
2. Using non-stick cooking oil, coat a muffin pan.
3. Heat the olive oil in a big non-stick skillet or pan over medium-high heat until it starts shimmering.
4. Add the broccoli and onion. Let it be for 3 minutes in the oven. Divide the vegetables equally among the four muffin cups.
5. Add the eggs, salt, garlic powder, and pepper. They can be poured over the vegetables in the muffin tins.
6. Bake for 15 to 17 minutes, or until the eggs are cooked through.

10.9 Shrimp Scampi

Preparation time-10 minutes| Cook time-15 minutes| Total time-25 minutes| Servings-2|Difficulty-Easy

Nutritional Facts- Calories: 345; Total Fat: 16; Total Carbs: 10g; Sugar: 3g; Fiber: 1g; Protein: 40g; Sodium: 424mg

Ingredients

- Half finely chopped onion
- One pound of peeled and tails removed shrimp
- Juice of one lemon
- Two tablespoons of extra-virgin olive oil
- Half chopped red bell pepper
- Three minced garlic cloves
- Zest of one lemon
- A pinch of freshly ground black pepper
- A quarter teaspoon of sea salt

Instructions

1. Heat the olive oil in a big non-stick pan over medium-high heat until it starts shimmering.
2. Add the red bell pepper and onion. Cook, stirring regularly, for around 6 minutes, or until tender.
3. Cook for around 5 minutes, or until the shrimp are yellow.
4. Add the garlic. Cook for 30 seconds while continuously stirring.
5. Stir in the zest and lemon juice, as well as the pepper and salt. Cook for 3 minutes on low heat.

10.10 Shrimp with Cinnamon Sauce

Preparation time-10 minutes| Cook time-10 minutes| Total time-20 minutes| Servings-2|Difficulty-Easy

Nutritional Facts- Calories: 270; Total Fat: 11g; Total Carbs: 4g; Sugar: <1g; Fiber: <1g; Protein: 39g; Sodium: 664mg

Ingredients

- One pound of peeled shrimp
- Half cup of no-salt-added chicken broth
- Half teaspoon of onion powder
- 1/8 teaspoon of freshly ground black pepper
- One tablespoon of extra-virgin olive oil
- One tablespoon of Dijon Mustard
- Half teaspoon of ground cinnamon
- A quarter teaspoon of sea salt

Instructions

1. Heat the olive oil in a big non-stick skillet or pan over medium-high heat until it starts shimmering.
2. Toss in the shrimp. Cook, stirring regularly, for around 4 minutes, or until the shrimp is opaque.
3. Whisk together the chicken broth, mustard, onion powder, salt, cinnamon, and pepper in a shallow cup. Pour this into the skillet or pan and fry, stirring regularly, for another 3 minutes.

10.11 Manhattan-Style Salmon Chowder

Preparation time-10 minutes| Cook time-15 minutes| Total time-25 minutes| Servings-2 |Difficulty-Easy

Nutritional Facts- Calories: 570; Total Fat: 42; Total Carbs: 55g; Sugar: 24g; Fiber: 16g; Protein: 41g; Sodium: 1,249mg

Ingredients

- Half chopped red bell pepper
- One(28-ounce) can of crushed tomatoes
- One cup of diced (Half-inch) sweet potatoes
- Two tablespoons of extra-virgin olive oil
- Half pound of skinless salmon, pin bones removed, chopped into half-inch pieces
- Three cups of no-salt-added chicken broth
- Half teaspoon of onion powder
- 1/8 teaspoon of freshly ground black pepper

- A quarter teaspoon of sea salt

Instructions

1. Heat the olive oil in a big pot over medium-high heat until it starts shimmering.
2. Add the salmon and red bell pepper. Cook, stirring regularly, for around 5 minutes, or until the fish is opaque and the bell pepper is tender.
3. Combine the chicken broth, tomatoes, onion powder, sweet potatoes, pepper, and salt in a large mixing bowl. Reduce the heat to medium-low and bring to a simmer. Cook, stirring regularly, for around 10 minutes, or until the sweet potatoes are tender.

10.12 Citrus Salmon on a Bed of Greens

Preparation time-10 minutes| Cook time-20 minutes| Total time-30 minutes| Servings-2|Difficulty-Easy

Nutritional Facts- Calories: 363; Total Fat: 25; Total Carbs: 3g; Sugar: <1g; Fiber: 1g; Protein: 34g; Sodium: 662mg

Ingredients

- One pound of salmon
- A quarter teaspoon of freshly ground black pepper
- Three cups of stemmed and chopped swiss chard
- Juice of one lemon
- Two tablespoons of extra-virgin olive oil
- Half teaspoon of sea salt
- Zest of one lemon
- Two minced garlic cloves

Instructions

1. Heat half of olive oil in a big non-stick skillet or pan over medium-high heat until it starts shimmering.
2. Half of the salt, pepper, and lemon zest are used to season the salmon.
3. Cook the salmon skin-side up in the skillet or pan for around 7 minutes or until the flesh is opaque. To crisp the skin, flip the salmon, and cook for another 3 to 4 minutes. Set out on a tray of aluminum foil tented around it.
4. Return the skillet or pan to the fire and drizzle in the remaining olive oil until it shimmers.
5. Add the Swiss chard. Cook, stirring regularly, for around 7 minutes, or until tender.
6. Add the garlic. Cook for 30 seconds while continuously stirring.
7. Add the remaining salt and a quarter teaspoon of pepper, along with the lemon juice. Let it be for 2 minutes in the oven
8. Serve the salmon with Swiss chard on the hand.

10.13 Salmon Ceviche

Preparation time-10 minutes plus 20 minutes resting time| Cook time-0 minutes| Total time-30 minutes| Servings-2|Difficulty-Easy

Nutritional Facts- Calories: 222; Total Fat: 14g; Total Carbs: 3g; Sugar: 2g; Fiber: <1g; Protein: 23g; Sodium: 288mg

Ingredients

- A quarter cup of freshly squeezed lime juice
- Two tablespoons of freshly chopped cilantro leaves
- Half pound salmon, skin and pins removed, cut into bite-size pieces
- One diced tomato
- One seeded and diced jalapeno pepper
- A quarter teaspoon of sea salt
- One tablespoon of extra-virgin olive oil

Instructions

1. Combine the lime juice and salmon in a medium mixing dish. Allow for a 20-minute marinade.
2. Combine the cilantro, tomatoes, olive oil, jalapeno, and salt in a mixing bowl.
3. Pour the cilantro mixture over the salmon, and then enjoy.

10.14 Rosemary-Lemon Cod

Preparation time-10 minutes| Cook time-11 minutes| Total time-21 minutes| Servings-2|Difficulty-Easy

Nutritional Facts- Calories: 246; Total Fat: 9g; Total Carbs: 1g; Sugar: <1g; Fiber: <1g; Protein: 39g; Sodium: 370mg

Ingredients

- One pound of Cod, skin, and bones removed, cut into four fillets
- A quarter teaspoon of freshly ground black pepper
- Juice of half a lemon
- One tablespoon of extra-virgin olive oil
- Half tablespoon of chopped fresh rosemary leaves
- A quarter teaspoon of sea salt

Instructions

1. Heat the olive oil in a big non-stick skillet or pan over medium-high heat until it starts shimmering.
2. Pepper, rosemary, and salt are used to season the fish. Cook the fish in the pan for 3 to 5 minutes on either hand or until opaque.
3. Cook for 1 minute after adding the lemon juice to the cod fillets.

10.15 Tuscan Chicken

Preparation time-5 minutes| Cook time-20 minutes| Total time-25 minutes| Servings-2|Difficulty-Easy

Nutritional Facts- Calories: 171; Total Fat: 11g; Total Carbs: 8g; Sugar: 4g; Fiber: 2g; Protein: 8g; Sodium: 743mg

Ingredients

- Half teaspoon of sea salt
- One teaspoon of garlic powder
- One chopped zucchini
- Four boneless and skinless chicken breast halves pounded to half-inch thick
- 1/8 teaspoon of freshly ground black pepper
- Two tablespoons of extra-virgin olive oil
- Two cups of cherry tomatoes
- A quarter cup of dry white wine
- Half cup of sliced green olives

Instructions

1. Using the pepper, salt, and garlic powder, season the chicken breasts.
2. Heat the olive oil in a big non-stick skillet or pan over medium-high heat until it starts shimmering. Cook for 7 to 10 minutes per hand or until the chicken reaches an internal temperature of 165°F. Remove the chicken from the pan and place it on a serving platter tented with foil.
3. Combine the tomatoes, zucchini, and olives in the same skillet or pan. Cook, stirring regularly, for around 4 minutes, or until the zucchini is soft.
4. Include the white wine and scrape some browned pieces off the bottom of the pan with a wooden spoon. One minute of simmering will be enough then, return the chicken to the plate, along with any juices that have gathered on the platter, and stir to combine the sauce and veggies.

10.16 Chicken Adobo

Preparation time-10 minutes| Cook time-15 minutes| Total time-25 minutes| Servings-2|Difficulty-Easy

Nutritional Facts- Calories: 698; Total Fat: 52g; Total Carbs: 11g; Sugar: 2g; Fiber: 2g; Protein: 46g; Sodium: 776mg

Ingredients

- One pound of skinless and boneless chicken breasts, cut into bite-size pieces
- Two tablespoons of low-sodium soy sauce
- Half teaspoon of onion powder
- 1/8 teaspoon of freshly ground black pepper

- One and a half tablespoons of extra-virgin olive oil
- One teaspoon of ground turmeric
- Half teaspoon of garlic powder
- A quarter teaspoon of sea salt

Instructions

1. Heat the olive oil in a big non-stick skillet or pan over medium-high heat until it starts shimmering. Then, add then chicken and turmeric to it.
2. Cook, stirring regularly, for 7 to 10 minutes, or until the chicken is cooked through. Then add the salt, garlic powder, soy sauce, onion powder, and pepper. Cook for 3 minutes, stirring occasionally.

10.17 Chicken Stir-Fry

Preparation time-15 minutes| Cook time-15 minutes| Total time-30 minutes| Servings-2|Difficulty-Easy

Nutritional Facts- Calories: 363; Total Fat: 22g; Total Carbs: 7g; Sugar: 2g; Fiber: 2g; Protein: 36g; Sodium: 993mg

Ingredients

- Three chopped scallions
- Half pound of boneless, skinless chicken breasts, cut into bite-size pieces
- Half tablespoon of toasted sesame seeds
- One and a half tablespoons of extra-virgin olive oil
- Half cup of broccoli florets
- Half cup of stir-fry sauce

Instructions

1. Heat the olive oil in a big non-stick skillet or pan over medium-high heat until it starts shimmering.
2. Add the broccoli, scallions, and chicken. Cook, stirring regularly, for 5 to 7 minutes, or until the chicken is fried and the vegetables are soft.
3. Add the stir-fry sauce to the pan. Cook, constantly stirring, for 5 minutes, or until the sauce has reduced.
4. If desired, sprinkle with sesame seeds.

10.18 Easy Chicken and Broccoli

Preparation time-10 minutes| Cook time-7 minutes| Total time-17 minutes| Servings-2|Difficulty-Easy

Nutritional Facts- Calories: 345; Total Fat: 14g; Total Carbs: 41g; Sugar: 1g; Fiber: 3g; Protein: 14g; Sodium: 276mg

Ingredients

- One pound of skinless and boneless chicken breasts, cut into bite-size pieces
- Half chopped onion
- 1/8 teaspoon of freshly ground black pepper
- One cup of cooked brown rice
- One and a half tablespoons of extra-virgin olive oil
- One cup of broccoli florets
- A quarter teaspoon of sea salt
- Two minced garlic cloves

Instructions

1. Heat the olive oil in a big non-stick skillet or pan over medium-high heat until it starts shimmering.
2. Add the chicken, salt, onion, broccoli, and pepper. Cook, stirring regularly, for around 7 minutes, or until the chicken is fried.
3. Afterward, garlic is to be added. Cook for 30 seconds while continuously stirring.
4. To serve, toss with the brown rice.

10.19 Chicken Sandwiches with Roasted Red Pepper Aioli

Preparation time-10 minutes| Cook time-10 minutes| Total time-20 minutes| Servings-2|Difficulty-Easy

Nutritional Facts- Calories: 318; Total Fat: 15g; Total Carbs: 36g; Sugar: 7g; Fiber: 6g; Protein: 13g; Sodium: 599mg

Ingredients

- Half pound of boneless, skinless chicken breasts, cut into four equal pieces and pounded ½ inch thick
- 1/8 teaspoon of freshly ground black pepper
- A quarter teaspoon of sea salt
- One tablespoon of extra-virgin olive oil
- Three roasted red pepper slices, divided
- Two whole-wheat buns
- Two tablespoons of anti-inflammatory mayonnaise

Instructions

1. Heat the olive oil in a big non-stick skillet or pan over medium-high heat until it starts shimmering.
2. Using pepper and salt, season the chicken. Cook for around 4 minutes per side in the pan or until the juices run free.

3. Combine the mayonnaise and two red pepper bits in a blender or food processor as the chicken cooks. Blend until entirely smooth.
4. Cover the buns with the remaining roasted red pepper slices and the sauce.
5. Add the chicken on top.

10.20 Turkey Scaloppine with Rosemary and Lemon Sauce

Preparation time-10 minutes| Cook time-15 minutes| Total time-25 minutes| Servings-2|Difficulty-Easy

Nutritional Facts- Calories: 188; Total Fat: 13g; Total Carbs: 8g; Sugar: 1g; Fiber: <1g; Protein: 10g; Sodium: 478mg

Ingredients

- Half teaspoon of sea salt, divided
- Two and a quarter pounds of boneless, skinless turkey breast cutlets, pounded 1/4 inch thick
- Juice of two lemons
- Half tablespoon of chopped fresh rosemary leaves
- Two tablespoons of whole-wheat flour
- 1/8 teaspoon of freshly ground black pepper
- Two tablespoons of extra-virgin olive oil, divided
- Zest of half a lemon

Instructions

1. Preheat the oven to 200 degrees Fahrenheit.
2. Using parchment paper, line a baking dish.
3. Whisk together the half teaspoon of salt, flour, and pepper in a shallow bowl.
4. Dip each cutlet in the flour and pat off any residue, working for one piece at a time.
5. Heat olive oil for each cutlet in the batch in a big skillet or pan over medium-high heat until it starts shimmering. Cook the cutlets for around 2 minutes per side in the hot oil. When the cutlets are finished, place them on the prepared baking sheet. Place the baking sheet in the oven to hold them warm until they're all finished.
6. Return the skillet or pan to the fire and let it be there until all of the cutlets are fried and warm. Add the lemon juice and zest to the skillet or pan. Scrape some browned pieces off the bottom of the skillet or pan with a wooden spoon.
7. Add the rosemary and salt. Cook, stirring continuously, for around 2 minutes, or until the sauce thickens.
8. Serve the cutlets with the sauce spooned over them.

10.21 Turkey Burgers with Ginger-Teriyaki Sauce and Pineapple

Preparation time-10 minutes| Cook time-10 minutes| Total time-20 minutes| Servings-2|Difficulty-Easy

Nutritional Facts- Calories: 366; Total Fat: 16g; Total Carbs: 23g; Sugar: 10g; Fiber: <1g; Protein: 34g; Sodium: 1,089mg

Ingredients

- A quarter teaspoon of sea salt
- One tablespoon of extra-virgin olive oil
- Two pineapple rings
- Half of pound ground turkey breast, formed into two patties
- A pinch of freshly ground black pepper
- Half cup of ginger-teriyaki sauce

Instructions

1. Using salt and pepper, season the turkey burgers.
2. Heat the olive oil in a big non-stick skillet or pan over medium-high heat until it starts shimmering.
3. Cook for about 7 minutes, rotating once until the burgers are cooked through and browned on both sides.
4. When the burgers are cooking, carry the teriyaki sauce to a boil in a small saucepan over medium-high heat, stirring continuously. Cook until the sauce thickens, around 1 to 2 minutes.
5. Serve the grilled burgers with the warmed sauce and pineapple rings on top.

10.22 Ground Turkey and Spinach Stir-Fry

Preparation time-10 minutes| Cook time-10 minutes| Total time-20 minutes| Servings-2|Difficulty-Easy

Nutritional Facts- Calories: 424; Total Fat: 20g; Total Carbs: 9g; Sugar: 3g; Fiber: 2g; Protein: 51g; Sodium: 1,016mg

Ingredients

- One pound of ground turkey breast
- One tablespoon of extra-virgin olive oil
- Half chopped onion
- Half cup of stir-fry sauce
- Two cups of fresh baby spinach

Instructions

1. Heat the olive oil in a big non-stick skillet or pan over medium-high heat until it starts shimmering.

2. Add the onion, turkey, and spinach. Cook, breaking up the turkey with a spoon for about 5 minutes before the meat is browned.

3. Add the stir-fry sauce to the pan. Cook, stirring continuously, for 3 to 4 minutes, or until it thickens. Then enjoy.

10.23 Pork Chops with Gingered Applesauce

Preparation time-10 minutes| Cook time-15 minutes| Total time-25 minutes| Servings-2|Difficulty-Easy

Nutritional Facts- Calories: 442; Total Fat: 10g; Total Carbs: 56g; Sugar: 44g; Fiber: 8g; Protein: 35g; Sodium: 301mg

Ingredients

- A quarter teaspoon of sea salt
- Three peeled, cored, and chopped apples
- Two thin-cut pork chops
- A pinch of freshly ground black pepper
- Two tablespoons of packed brown sugar
- Half tablespoon of grated fresh ginger
- Two tablespoons of water

Instructions

1. Preheat the oven to 425 degrees Fahrenheit.
2. Salt and pepper the pork chops and place them on a rimmed baking sheet. Bake for 15 minutes or until an instant-read meat thermometer detects a temperature of 165°F.
3. Meanwhile, add the apples, water, brown sugar, and ginger in a big pot over medium-high heat. Cook, covered, for around 10 minutes, or until the apples have softened into a gravy, stirring periodically.

10.24 Macadamia-Dusted Pork Cutlets

Preparation time-10 minutes| Cook time-10 minutes| Total time-20 minutes| Servings-2|Difficulty-Easy

Nutritional Facts- Calories: 437; Total Fat: 33g; Total Carbs: 6g; Sugar: 3g; Fiber: 3g; Protein: 33g; Sodium: 309mg

Ingredients

- Half teaspoon of sea salt, divided
- A quarter cup of macadamia nuts, pulsed in a blender or food processor to form a powder
- One tablespoon of extra-virgin olive oil
- Half of one (1-pound) pork tenderloin, cut into 1/2-inch slices and pounded uniformly thin
- 1/8 teaspoon of freshly ground black pepper, divided
- Half cup of full-fat coconut milk

Instructions

1. Preheat the oven to 400 degrees Fahrenheit.
2. Half of salt and pepper are used to season the pork chops.
3. Combine the remaining half of salt, the macadamia nut powder, and the remaining pepper in a small bowl.
4. In a separate shallow bowl, mix together the coconut milk and olive oil.
5. Dip the pork in the macadamia nut powder and then into the coconut milk. Place it on a baking sheet with a bottom. Repeat for the rest of the pork slices.
6. Bake the pork for around 10 minutes or before an instant-read meat thermometer, detects an internal temperature of 165°F.

10.25 Lamb Meatballs with Garlic Aioli

Preparation time-15 minutes| Cook time-15 minutes| Total time-30 minutes| Servings-2|Difficulty-Easy

Nutritional Facts- Calories: 445; Total Fat: 23g; Total Carbs: 10g; Sugar: 2g; Fiber: 1g; Protein: 48g; Sodium:574mg

Ingredients

- One tablespoon of dried rosemary leaves
- Half teaspoon of onion powder
- A quarter teaspoon of sea salt
- A quarter cup of garlic aioli
- One pound of ground lamb
- Half tablespoon of dried oregano
- Half teaspoon of garlic powder
- 1/8 of freshly ground black pepper

Instructions

1. Preheat the oven to 400 degrees Fahrenheit.
2. Combine the lamb, oregano, rosemary, garlic powder, onion powder, pepper, and salt in a big mixing bowl. Place the mixture on a rimmed baking sheet and roll it into ten 3/4-inch balls.
3. Bake for 15 minutes or until an instant-read meat thermometer detects 145°F internal temperature.
4. Serve with aioli on the side.

10.26 Beef Flank Steak Tacos with Guacamole

Preparation time-10 minutes| Cook time-14 minutes| Total time-24 minutes| Servings-2|Difficulty-Easy

Nutritional Facts- Calories: 717; Total Fat: 52g; Total Carbs: 12g; Sugar: 8g; Fiber: 1g; Protein: 54g; Sodium: 590mg

Ingredients

- Three tablespoons of extra-virgin olive oil, divided
- Half chopped jalapeño pepper
- A quarter teaspoon of sea salt
- Half cup of guacamole
- Two tablespoons of fresh cilantro leaves
- Two minced garlic cloves
- One pound of beef flank steak
- A pinch of freshly ground black pepper

Instructions

1. Combine the cilantro, two tablespoons of olive oil, ginger, and jalapeno in a blender or food processor. To render a paste, pulse 10 to 20 times (1 second). One tablespoon of the paste should be set aside, and the rest should be poured over the flank steak. Allow for a 5-minute rest period.
2. Heat the remaining one tablespoon of olive oil in a big skillet or pan over medium-high heat until it starts shimmering.
3. Toss in the steak. Cook for around 7 minutes per hand or before an instant-read meat thermometer reads 125°F internal temperature.
4. Allow the steak to rest for 5 minutes on a cutting board. Cut it into half-inch-thick slices against the grain.
5. Toss the slices with the reserved dressing of herb paste in a medium dish.
6. Serve with guacamole on the side.

10.27 Beef and Broccoli Stir-Fry

Preparation time-10 minutes| Cook time-10 minutes| Total time-20 minutes| Servings-2|Difficulty-Easy

Nutritional Facts- Calories: 302; Total Fat: 17g; Total Carbs: 4g; Sugar: 2g; Fiber: 1g; Protein: 33g; Sodium: 523mg

Ingredients

- Half pound of flank steak, sliced against the grain into ½-inch strips
- Half cup of sugar snap peas
- Two tablespoons of stir-fry sauce
- One tablespoon of extra-virgin olive oil
- Half cup of broccoli florets
- Half chopped zucchini

Instructions

1. Heat the olive oil in a big non-stick skillet or pan over medium-high heat until it starts shimmering.
2. Cook for 5 to 7 minutes, stirring regularly until the beef is browned. With a slotted spoon, remove the chicken and place it on a platter.
3. Add the sugar snap peas, broccoli, and zucchini. Cook, stirring regularly, for around 5 minutes, or until the veggies are crisp-tender.
4. Toss the beef back into the pan. Add the stir-fry sauce to the pan. Cook for 3 minutes, occasionally stirring, until thoroughly heated.

10.28 Beef and Bell Pepper Fajitas

Preparation time-5 minutes| Cook time-10 minutes| Total time-15 minutes| Servings-2 |Difficulty-Easy

Nutritional Facts- Calories: 470; Total Fat: 25g; Total Carbs: 12g; Sugar: 6g; Fiber: 3g; Protein: 49g; Sodium: 722mg

Ingredients

- One pound of flank steak, cut against the grain into 1/2-inch strips
- Half sliced onion
- One and a half tablespoons of extra-virgin olive oil
- One sliced green bell peppers
- Half cup of store-bought salsa
- A quarter teaspoon of sea salt
- Half teaspoon of garlic powder

Instructions

1. Heat the olive oil in a big non-stick skillet or pan over medium-high heat until it starts shimmering.
2. Add bell peppers, beef, and onion. Cook, stirring regularly, for around 6 minutes, or until the beef browns.
3. Stir the garlic powder, salsa, and salt. Cook for 3 minutes, stirring occasionally.

10.29 Hamburger with Pub Sauce

Preparation time-10 minutes| Cook time-10 minutes| Total time-20 minutes| Servings-2|Difficulty-Easy

Nutritional Facts- Calories: 333; Total Fat: 18g; Total Carbs: 13g; Sugar: 7g; Fiber: <1g; Protein: 31g; Sodium: 968mg

Ingredients

- A quarter teaspoon of sea salt
- A quarter cup of garlic aioli
- Half pound of extra-lean ground beef, formed into four patties

- A pinch of freshly ground black pepper
- One and a half tablespoons of low-sodium soy sauce
- One tablespoon of chopped fresh chives
- One tablespoon of brown sugar

Instructions

1. Season the patties with salt and pepper.
2. Cook the patties in a wide skillet or pan over medium-high heat for around 5 minutes per hand or until an instant-read meat thermometer registers an internal temperature of 145°F.
3. In a bit of bowl, mix together the soy sauce, brown sugar, aioli, and chives while the hamburgers are cooking.
4. Serve the aioli with the hamburgers, as well as something else that appeals to the palate.

10.30 Quinoa-Stuffed Collard Rolls

Preparation time-15 minutes| Cook time-0 minutes| Total time-15 minutes| Servings-2|Difficulty-Easy

Nutritional Facts- Calories: 321; Total Fat: 13g; Total Carbs: 18g; Sugar: 6g; Fiber: 1g; Protein: 23g; Sodium: 768mg

Ingredients

- Half cup of quinoa
- A quarter cup of pecans
- Half diced small onion
- One shredded carrot
- Half teaspoon of ground sage
- One teaspoon of sea salt
- One and a half cups of vegetable broth, divided
- Half a bunch of collard greens washed with stems removed
- Half tablespoon of grapeseed oil
- A quarter of chopped mushrooms
- One clove of garlic
- Half teaspoon of dried oregano

Instructions

1. Bring one cup of broth and the quinoa to a boil in a medium saucepan over medium-high flame. Reduce the heat to a minimum, cover, and cook for 20 minutes, stirring occasionally. Allow cooling for around 5 minutes after fluffing with a fork.
2. Preheat oven to 350 degrees Fahrenheit.
3. A big pot of water should be brought to a boil. 2 minutes after, add the collard greens, blanch them. Then remove from the heat, rinse with cool water and drain.

4. In a small dry sauté pan, toast the pecans over medium heat until fragrant and beginning to brown slightly.
5. Chop the nuts coarsely.
6. In a big sauté pan, heat the oil over medium heat. Sauté the onion until it is transparent. Sauté for 2 minutes after adding the mushrooms. Sauté for 3 minutes with the garlic, sage, carrots, and oregano.
7. Combine the pecans, quinoa, and salt in a mixing bowl.
8. Fill a collard leaf with a large scoop of filling. Burrito-style roll the leaf and put the seam down in a square baking dish.
9. Continue before you've used up enough of the collards and filling. Cover the rolls with foil and bake for 25 minutes with the remaining half cup of broth.

Chapter 11-Dinner Recipes

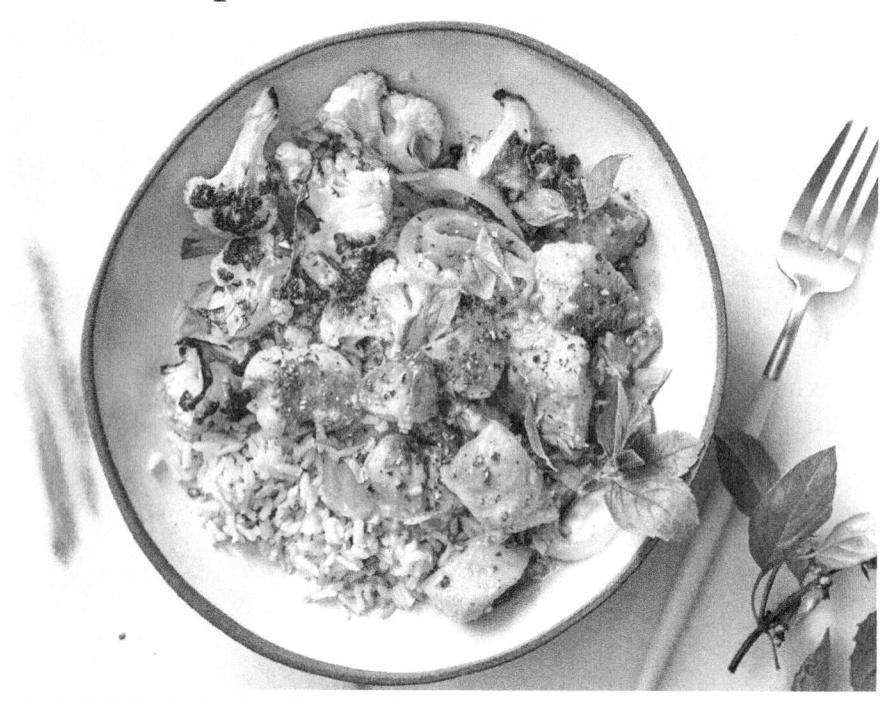

11.1 Whole-Wheat Pasta with Tomato-Basil Sauce

Preparation time-15 minutes| Cook time-10 minutes| Total time-25 minutes| Servings-2|Difficulty-Easy

Nutritional Facts- Calories: 330; Total Fat: 8g; Total Carbs: 56g; Sugar: 24g; Fiber: 17g; Protein: 14g; Sodium: 1,000mg

Ingredients

- Half minced onion
- One(28-ounce) can of crushed tomatoes, undrained
- 1/8 teaspoon of freshly ground black pepper
- Half of one (8-ounce) package whole-wheat pasta
- One tablespoon of extra-virgin olive oil
- Three minced garlic cloves
- A quarter teaspoon of sea salt
- Two tablespoons of chopped basil leaves

Instructions

1. Heat the olive oil in a big pot over medium-high heat until it starts shimmering.
2. Toss in the onion. Cook, stirring regularly, for around 5 minutes, or until tender.
3. Garlic can be included now. Cook for 30 seconds while continuously stirring.
4. Add the salt, tomatoes, and pepper. Bring to a low boil, then reduce to low heat. Reduce the heat to medium and simmer, stirring periodically, for 5 minutes.

5. Remove the pan from the heat and add the basil. Toss the spaghetti with the sauce.

11.2 Tofu and Spinach Sauté

Preparation time-10 minutes| Cook time-10 minutes| Total time-20 minutes| Servings-2|Difficulty-Easy

Nutritional Facts- Calories: 128; Total Fat: 10g; Total Carbs: 7g; Sugar: 3g; Fiber: 2g; Protein: 6g; Sodium: 266mg

Ingredients

- Half chopped onion
- Four ounces of tofu
- Juice of half an orange
- One tablespoon of extra-virgin olive oil
- Two cups of fresh baby spinach
- Two minced garlic cloves
- Zest of half an orange
- A pinch of freshly ground black pepper
- Half teaspoon of sea salt

Instructions

1. Heat the olive oil in a big skillet or pan over medium-high heat until it starts shimmering.
2. Add the spinach, onion, and tofu. Cook, stirring regularly, for around 5 minutes, or until the onion is tender.
3. Garlic can be included now. Cook for 30 seconds while continuously stirring.
4. Add the orange juice, salt, orange zest, and pepper. Cook for 3 minutes, occasionally stirring, until thoroughly heated.

11.3 Sweet Potato Curry with Spinach

Preparation time-10 minutes| Cook time-20 minutes| Total time-30 minutes| Servings-2|Difficulty-Easy

Nutritional Facts- Calories: 314; Total Fat: 11g; Total Carbs: 50g; Sugar: 14g; Fiber: 9g; Protein: 8g; Sodium: 400mg

Ingredients

- Half chopped onion
- Two cups of fresh baby spinach
- Half cup of lite coconut milk
- One tablespoon of extra-virgin olive oil
- Two cups of cubed peeled sweet potato
- Two cups of no-salt-added vegetable broth

- One tablespoon of curry powder
- A pinch of freshly ground black pepper
- A quarter teaspoon of sea salt

Instructions

1. Heat the olive oil in a big pot over medium-high heat until it starts shimmering.
2. Toss in the onion. Cook, stirring regularly, for around 5 minutes, or until tender.
3. Add the spinach, sweet potato, vegetable broth, curry powder, coconut milk, salt, and pepper to the sweet potato mixture. Reduce the heat to medium-low and bring to a simmer. Cook, stirring regularly, for around 15 minutes, or until the sweet potatoes are tender.

11.4 Buckwheat Noodles with Peanut Sauce

Preparation time-20 minutes| Cook time-0 minutes| Total time-20 minutes| Servings-2|Difficulty-Easy

Nutritional Facts- Calories: 388; Total Fat: 18g; Total Carbs: 51g; Sugar: 4g; Fiber: 8g; Protein: 16g; Sodium: 542mg

Ingredients

- Half cup of peanut sauce
- Half of one (8-ounce) package of buckwheat noodles, cooked according to package directions and drained
- Two tablespoons of chopped fresh cilantro leaves
- Three scallions, white and green parts, thinly sliced diagonally
- Two tablespoons of chopped peanuts

Instructions

1. Toss the buckwheat noodles with the peanut sauce in a big mixing bowl to cover.
2. Serve with peanuts, cilantro, and scallions as garnish.

11.5 Kale Frittata

Preparation time-10 minutes| Cook time-17 minutes| Total time-27 minutes| Servings-2|Difficulty-Easy

Nutritional Facts- Calories: 231; Total Fat: 17g; Total Carbs: 9g; Sugar: <1g; Fiber: 1g; Protein: 14g; Sodium: 387mg

Ingredients

- One tablespoon of extra-virgin olive oil
- Two cups of stemmed and chopped kale
- Two minced garlic cloves
- Four eggs
- A quarter teaspoon of sea salt

- 1/8 teaspoon of freshly ground black pepper
- One tablespoon of sunflower seeds

Instructions

1. Preheat the broiler to the highest setting.
2. Heat the olive oil in a big ovenproof skillet or pan over medium-high heat until it starts shimmering.
3. Toss in the kale. Cook, stirring regularly, for around 5 minutes, or until tender.
4. Garlic can be included now. Cook for 30 seconds while continuously stirring.
5. Whisk the salt, eggs, and pepper in a medium mixing bowl. Pour them over the kale with care. Turn the heat down to medium.
6. Cook for 3 minutes, or until the eggs are hardened around the outside. Carefully draw the eggs away from the skillet or pan's sides with a rubber spatula, then tilt the pan to allow the uncooked eggs to run into the edges. Cook for 3 minutes, or until the edges are set.
7. Sunflower seeds can be sprinkled on top. Preheat the broiler and cook the pan for 3 to 5 minutes, or until puffed and brown. To eat, cut into wedges.

11.6 Black Bean Chili with Garlic and Tomatoes

Preparation time-10 minutes| Cook time-20 minutes| Total time-30 minutes| Servings-2|Difficulty-Easy

Nutritional Facts- Calories: 481; Total Fat: 10g; Total Carbs: 80g; Sugar: 14g; Fiber: 21g; Protein: 25g; Sodium: 278mg

Ingredients

- Half chopped onion
- One (14-ounce) can of black beans, drained
- One tablespoon of extra-virgin olive oil
- One (28-ounce) can of chopped tomatoes, undrained
- Half tablespoon of chili powder
- A quarter teaspoon of sea salt
- Half teaspoon of garlic powder

Instructions

1. Heat the olive oil in a big pot over medium-high heat until it starts shimmering.
2. Toss in the onion. Cook, stirring regularly, for around 5 minutes, or until tender.
3. Add the black beans, tomatoes, garlic powder, chili powder, and salt. Bring to a low boil, then reduce to low heat. Reduce the heat to medium and simmer, stirring regularly, for 15 minutes.

11.7 Mushroom Pesto Burgers

Preparation time-5 minutes| Cook time-20 minutes| Total time-25 minutes| Servings-2|Difficulty-Easy

Nutritional Facts- Calories: 339; Total Fat: 23; Total Carbs: 26g; Sugar: 6g; Fiber: 5g; Protein: 12g; Sodium: 278mg

Ingredients

- Half cup of spinach pesto
- Two portobello mushroom caps stemmed, gills removed
- Two onion slices
- Two whole-wheat hamburger buns
- Two tomato slices

Instructions

1. Preheat the oven to 400 degrees Fahrenheit.
2. Brush all sides of the mushroom caps with pesto and arrange them on a rimmed baking sheet. Bake for 15 to 20 minutes, or until soft.
3. On the buns, layer the tomatoes, mushrooms, and onions.

11.8 Egg Salad Cups

Preparation time-15 minutes| Cook time-0 minutes| Total time-15 minutes| Servings-2|Difficulty-Easy

Nutritional Facts- Calories: 190; Total Fat: 14; Total Carbs: 6g; Sugar: 2g; Fiber: <1g; Protein: 11g; Sodium: 477mg

Ingredients

- A quarter of finely chopped red bell pepper
- Half teaspoon of Dijon mustard
- Four hard-boiled eggs, peeled and chopped
- Two tablespoons of anti-inflammatory mayonnaise
- A quarter teaspoon of sea salt
- Two large lettuce leaves
- A pinch of freshly ground black pepper

Instructions

1. Combine the red bell pepper, eggs, mayonnaise, salt, mustard, and pepper in a big mixing cup. To merge, softly mix all together.
2. Fill the lettuce leaves with the mixture.

11.9 Shrimp with Spicy Spinach

Preparation time-10 minutes| Cook time-15 minutes| Total time-25 minutes| Servings-2|Difficulty-Easy

Nutritional Facts- Calories: 317; Total Fat: 16; Total Carbs: 7g; Sugar: 3g; Fiber: <1g; Protein: 38g; Sodium: 911mg

Ingredients

- One pound of peeled shrimp
- Two cups of fresh baby spinach
- A quarter cup of freshly squeezed orange juice
- A pinch of freshly ground black pepper
- Two tablespoons of extra-virgin olive oil, divided
- Half teaspoon of sea salt, divided
- Three minced garlic cloves
- Half tablespoon of sriracha sauce

Instructions

1. Heat one tablespoon of olive oil in a big non-stick skillet or pan over medium-high heat until it starts shimmering.
2. Add half of the salt and the shrimp. Cook, stirring regularly, for around 4 minutes, or until the shrimp are pink. Place the shrimp on a plate and cover with aluminum foil to keep them soft.
3. Return the skillet or pan to heat and add the remaining one tablespoon of olive oil, constantly stirring until it shimmers.
4. Toss in the spinach. Cook for 3 minutes, stirring occasionally.
5. Garlic can be included now. Cook for 30 seconds while continuously stirring.
6. Whisk together the Sriracha, orange juice, some salt, and pepper in a shallow bowl. Cook for 3 minutes after adding this to the spinach.
7. Serve the shrimp with a side of spinach.

11.10 Pan-Seared Scallops with Lemon-Ginger Vinaigrette

Preparation time-10 minutes| Cook time-7 minutes| Total time-17 minutes| Servings-2|Difficulty-Easy

Nutritional Facts- Calories: 280; Total Fat: 16; Total Carbs: 5g; Sugar: <1g; Fiber: 0g; Protein: 29g; Sodium: 508mg

Ingredients

- One pound of sea scallops
- One tablespoon of extra-virgin olive oil
- A quarter teaspoon of sea salt
- Two tablespoons of lemon-ginger vinaigrette

- A pinch of freshly ground black pepper

Instructions

1. Heat the olive oil in a big non-stick skillet or pan over medium-high heat until it starts shimmering.
2. Add the scallops to the skillet or pan after seasoning them with pepper and salt. Cook for 3 minutes per side or until the fish is only opaque.
3. Serve with a dollop of vinaigrette on top.

11.11 Roasted Salmon and Asparagus

Preparation time-5 minutes| Cook time-15 minutes| Total time-20 minutes| Servings-2|Difficulty-Easy

Nutritional Facts- Calories: 308; Total Fat: 18g; Total Carbs: 5g; Sugar: 2g; Fiber: 2g; Protein: 36g; Sodium: 542mg

Ingredients

- One tablespoon of extra-virgin olive oil
- One pound of salmon, cut into two fillets
- Zest and slices of half lemon
- Half pound of asparagus spears, trimmed
- One teaspoon of sea salt, divided
- 1/8 teaspoon of freshly cracked black pepper

Instructions

1. Preheat the oven to 425 degrees Fahrenheit.
2. Stir the asparagus with half of salt and olive oil. At the base of a roasting tray, spread in a continuous sheet.
3. With salt and pepper the salmon is to be seasoned. Place the asparagus on top of the skin-side down.
4. Lemon zest should be sprinkled over the asparagus and salmon, and lemon slices should be placed over the top.
5. Roast for around 15 minutes, or until the flesh of the fish is opaque, in a preheated oven.

11.12 Orange and Maple-Glazed Salmon

Preparation time-15 minutes| Cook time-15 minutes| Total time-30 minutes| Servings-2|Difficulty-Easy

Nutritional Facts- Calories: 297; Total Fat: 11; Total Carbs: 18g; Sugar: 15g; Fiber: <1g; Protein: 34g; Sodium: 528mg

Ingredients

- Zest of one orange
- One tablespoon of low-sodium soy sauce

- Two (4- to 6-ounce) salmon fillets, pin bones removed
- Juice of one orange
- Two tablespoons of pure maple syrup
- One teaspoon of garlic powder

Instructions

1. Preheat the oven to 400 degrees Fahrenheit.
2. Whisk together the orange juice and zest, soy sauce, maple syrup, and garlic powder in a little shallow bowl.
3. Place the salmon parts in the dish flesh-side down. Allow 10 minutes for marinating.
4. Place the salmon on a rimmed baking dish, skin-side up, and bake for 15 minutes, or until the flesh is opaque.

11.13 Cod with Ginger and Black Beans

Preparation time-10 minutes| Cook time-15 minutes| Total time-25 minutes| Servings-2|Difficulty-Easy

Nutritional Facts- Calories: 419; Total Fat: 2g; Total Carbs: 33g; Sugar: 1g; Fiber: 8g; Protein: 50g; Sodium: 605mg

Ingredients

- Two (6-ounce) cod fillets
- Half teaspoon of sea salt, divided
- Three minced garlic cloves
- Two tablespoons of chopped fresh cilantro leaves
- One tablespoon of extra-virgin olive oil
- Half tablespoon of grated fresh ginger
- Two tablespoons of freshly ground black pepper
- Half of one (14-ounce) can of black beans, drained

Instructions

1. Heat the olive oil in a big non-stick skillet or pan over medium-high heat until it starts shimmering.
2. Half of the salt, ginger, and pepper are used to season the fish. Cook for around 4 minutes per side in the hot oil until the fish is opaque. Remove the cod from the pan and place it on a platter with aluminum foil tented over it.
3. Add the garlic to the skillet or pan and return it to the heat. Cook for 30 seconds while continuously stirring.
4. Add the black beans and the remaining salt. Cook, stirring regularly, for 5 minutes.
5. Add the cilantro and serve the black beans on top of the cod.

11.14 Halibut Curry

Preparation time-10 minutes| Cook time-10 minutes| Total time-20 minutes| Servings-2|Difficulty-Easy

Nutritional Facts- Calories: 429; Total Fat: 47g; Total Carbs: 5g; Sugar: <1g; Fiber: <1g; Protein: 27g; Sodium: 507mg

Ingredients

- One teaspoon of ground turmeric
- One pound of halibut, skin, and bones removed, cut into 1-inch pieces
- Half of one (14-ounce) can lite coconut milk
- 1/8 teaspoon of freshly ground black pepper
- One tablespoon of extra-virgin olive oil
- One teaspoon of curry powder
- Two cups of no-salt-added chicken broth
- A quarter teaspoon of sea salt

Instructions

1. Heat the olive oil in a big non-stick skillet or pan over medium-high heat until it starts shimmering.
2. Add the curry powder and turmeric to a bowl. To bloom the spices, cook for 2 minutes, stirring continuously.
3. Stir in the halibut, coconut milk, chicken broth, pepper, and salt. Reduce the heat to medium-low and bring to a simmer. Cook, stirring regularly, for 6 to 7 minutes, or until the fish is opaque.

11.15 Chicken Cacciatore

Preparation time-10 minutes| Cook time-20 minutes| Total time-30 minutes| Servings-2|Difficulty-Easy

Nutritional Facts- Calories: 305; Total Fat: 11g; Total Carbs: 34g; Sugar: 23g; Fiber: 13g; Protein: 19g; Sodium: 1,171mg

Ingredients

- One pound of skinless and boneless chicken breasts, cut into bite-size pieces
- A quarter cup of black olives, chopped
- Half teaspoon of onion powder
- A pinch of freshly ground black pepper
- One tablespoon of extra-virgin olive oil
- One(28-ounce) can of crushed tomatoes, drained
- Half teaspoon of garlic powder
- A quarter teaspoon of sea salt

Instructions

1. Heat the olive oil in a big non-stick skillet or pan over medium-high heat until it starts shimmering.
2. Cook, stirring regularly, for 7 to 10 minutes, until the chicken is browned.
3. Add the tomatoes, garlic powder, olives, salt, onion powder, then pepper, and stir to combine. Cook, stirring regularly, for 10 minutes.

11.16 Chicken and Bell Pepper Sauté

Preparation time-15 minutes| Cook time-15 minutes| Total time-30 minutes| Servings-2|Difficulty-Easy

Nutritional Facts- Calories: 179; Total Fat: 13g; Total Carbs: 6g; Sugar: 3g; Fiber: 1g; Protein: 10g; Sodium: 265mg

Ingredients

- One chopped bell pepper
- One pound of skinless and boneless chicken breasts, cut into bite-size pieces
- One and a half tablespoons of extra-virgin olive oil
- Half chopped onion
- Three minced garlic cloves
- 1/8 teaspoon of freshly ground black pepper
- A quarter teaspoon of sea salt

Instructions

1. Heat the olive oil in a big non-stick skillet or pan over medium-high heat until it starts shimmering.
2. Add the onion, red bell pepper, and chicken. Cook, stirring regularly, for 10 minutes.
3. Stir in the salt, garlic, and pepper in a mixing bowl. Cook for 30 seconds while continuously stirring.

11.17 Chicken Salad Sandwiches

Preparation time-15 minutes| Cook time-0 minutes| Total time-15 minutes| Servings-2|Difficulty-Easy

Nutritional Facts- Calories: 315; Total Fat: 9g; Total Carbs: 30g; Sugar: 6g; Fiber: 4g; Protein: 28g; Sodium:677mg

Ingredients

- Two tablespoons of anti-inflammatory mayonnaise
- One tablespoon of chopped fresh tarragon leaves
- One cup of chopped, cooked, skinless chicken from a rotisserie chicken
- Half minced red bell pepper
- One teaspoon of Dijon mustard

- Four slices of whole-wheat bread
- A quarter teaspoon of sea salt

Instructions

1. Combine the chicken, red bell pepper, mayonnaise, mustard, tarragon, and salt in a medium mixing bowl.
2. Spread on four pieces of bread and top it with the remaining bread.

11.18 Rosemary Chicken

Preparation time-10 minutes| Cook time-20 minutes| Total time-30 minutes| Servings-2|Difficulty-Easy

Nutritional Facts- Calories: 389; Total Fat: 20g; Total Carbs: 1g; Sugar: 0g; Fiber: <1g; Protein: 49g; Sodium: 381mg

Ingredients

- One tablespoon of extra-virgin olive oil
- One pound of chicken breast tenders
- One tablespoon of chopped fresh rosemary leaves
- 1/8 teaspoon of freshly ground black pepper
- A quarter teaspoon of sea salt

Instructions

1. Preheat the oven to 425 degrees Fahrenheit.
2. Place the chicken tenders on a baking sheet with a rim. Sprinkle with salt, rosemary, and pepper after brushing them with olive oil.
3. For 15 to 20 minutes, keep in the oven, just before the juices run clear.

11.19 Gingered Turkey Meatballs

Preparation time-10 minutes| Cook time-10 minutes| Total time-20 minutes| Servings-2|Difficulty-Easy

Nutritional Facts- Calories: 408; Total Fat: 26g; Total Carbs: 4g; Sugar: 1g; Fiber: 1g; Protein: 47g; Sodium: 426mg

Ingredients

- Half cup of shredded cabbage
- Half tablespoon of grated fresh ginger
- Half teaspoon of onion powder
- One pound of ground turkey
- Two tablespoons of chopped fresh cilantro leaves
- Half teaspoon of garlic powder
- A quarter teaspoon of sea salt

- One tablespoon of olive oil
- A pinch of freshly ground black pepper

Ingredients

1. Combine the cabbage, turkey, cilantro, ginger, onion powder, garlic powder, pepper, and salt in a big mixing bowl. Mix well. Make ten 3/4-inch meatballs out of the turkey mixture.
2. Heat the olive oil in a big non-stick skillet or pan over medium-high heat until it starts shimmering.
3. Cook for about 10 minutes, rotating the meatballs while they brown and you are done.

11.20 Turkey and Kale Sauté

Preparation time-10 minutes| Cook time-10 minutes| Total time-20 minutes| Servings-2|Difficulty-Easy

Nutritional Facts- Calories: 413; Total Fat: 20g; Total Carbs: 7g; Sugar: <1g; Fiber: 1g; Protein: 50g; Sodium: 358mg

Ingredients

- One pound of ground turkey breast
- Half chopped onion
- Half teaspoon of sea salt
- Three minced garlic cloves
- One tablespoon of extra-virgin olive oil
- One cup of stemmed and chopped kale
- One tablespoon of fresh thyme leaves
- A pinch of freshly ground black pepper

Instructions

1. Heat the olive oil in a big non-stick skillet or pan over medium-high heat until it starts shimmering.
2. Add the turkey, onion, kale, thyme, pepper, and salt. Cook, crumbling the turkey with a spoon until it browns, for about 5 minutes.
3. Garlic can be included now. Cook for 30 minutes while continuously stirring.

11.21 Turkey with Bell Peppers and Rosemary

Preparation time-10 minutes| Cook time-10 minutes| Total time-20 minutes| Servings-2|Difficulty-Easy

Nutritional Facts- Calories: 303; Total Fat: 14g; Total Carbs: 15g; Sugar: 10g; Fiber: 2g; Protein: 30g; Sodium: 387mg

Ingredients

- One chopped red bell peppers
- One pound of boneless, skinless turkey breasts, cut into bite-size pieces

- A quarter teaspoon of sea salt
- Two minced garlic cloves
- Two tablespoons of extra-virgin olive oil
- Half chopped onion
- One tablespoon of chopped fresh rosemary leaves
- A pinch of freshly ground black pepper

Instructions

1. Heat the olive oil in a big non-stick skillet or pan over medium-high heat until it starts shimmering.
2. Add the onion, red bell peppers, turkey, salt, and pepper. Cook, stirring regularly, for 7 to 10 minutes, or until the turkey is cooked and the veggies are soft.
3. Garlic can be included now. Cook for an additional 30 seconds, stirring continuously.

11.22 Mustard and Rosemary Pork Tenderloin

Preparation time-10 minutes| Cook time-15 minutes| Total time-25 minutes| Servings-2|Difficulty-Easy

Nutritional Facts- Calories: 362; Total Fat: 18g; Total Carbs: 5g; Sugar: <1g; Fiber: 2g; Protein: 2g; Sodium: 515mg

Ingredients

- Two tablespoons of Dijon mustard
- Two tablespoons of fresh rosemary leaves
- A quarter teaspoon of sea salt
- Half of one (1½-pound) pork tenderloin
- A quarter cup of fresh parsley leaves
- Three garlic cloves
- One and a half tablespoons of extra-virgin olive oil
- 1/8 teaspoon of freshly ground black pepper

Instructions

1. Preheat the oven to 400 degrees Fahrenheit.
2. Combine the mustard, parsley, garlic, olive oil, rosemary, pepper, and salt in a blender or food processor. Pulse 20 times in 1-second intervals before a paste emerges. Rub the tenderloin with the paste and place it on a rimmed baking sheet.
3. Bake the pork for around 15 minutes or until an instant-read meat thermometer, reads 165°F.
4. Allow resting for 5 minutes before slicing and serving.

11.23 Thin-Cut Pork Chops with Mustardy Kale

Preparation time-10 minutes| Cook time-15 minutes| Total time-25 minutes| Servings-2|Difficulty-Easy

Nutritional Facts- Calories: 504; Total Fat: 39g; Total Carbs: 10g; Sugar: <1g; Fiber: 2g; Protein: 28g; Sodium: 755mg

Ingredients

- One teaspoon of sea salt, divided
- Two tablespoons Dijon mustard, divided
- Half finely chopped red onion
- One tablespoon of apple cider vinegar
- Two thin-cut pork chops
- 1/8 teaspoon of freshly ground black pepper, divided
- One and a half tablespoons of extra-virgin olive oil
- Two cups of stemmed and chopped kale

Instructions

1. Preheat the oven to 425 degrees Fahrenheit.
2. Half of salt and pepper are used to season the pork chops. Place them on a rimmed baking sheet and spread one tablespoon of mustard over them. Bake for 15 minutes or until an instant-read meat thermometer detects a temperature of 165°F.
3. When the pork cooks, heat the olive oil in a big non-stick skillet or pan over medium-high heat until it starts shimmering.
4. Add the red onion and kale. Cook, stirring regularly, for around 7 minutes, or until the veggies soften.
5. Whisk together the remaining one tablespoon of mustard, the remaining half salt, the cider vinegar, and the remaining pepper in a wide mixing bowl. Toss with the kale. Cook for 2 minutes, stirring occasionally.

11.24 Beef Tenderloin with Savory Blueberry Sauce

Preparation time-10 minutes| Cook time-15 minutes| Total time-25 minutes| Servings-2|Difficulty-Easy

Nutritional Facts- Calories: 554; Total Fat: 32g; Total Carbs: 14g; Sugar: 8g; Fiber: 2g; Protein: 50g; Sodium: 632mg

Ingredients

- One teaspoon of sea salt, divided
- Two tablespoons of extra-virgin olive oil
- A quarter cup of tawny port
- One and a half tablespoons of very cold butter, cut into pieces

- Two beef tenderloin filets, about 3/4 inch thick
- 1/8 teaspoon of freshly ground black pepper, divided
- One finely minced shallot
- One cup of fresh blueberries

Instructions

1. Half salt and pepper are to be used to season the beef.
2. Heat the olive oil in a big skillet or pan over medium-high heat until it starts shimmering.
3. Add the seasoned steaks to the pan. Cook for 5 minutes per side or until an instant-read meat thermometer detects an internal temperature of 130°F. Set aside on a platter of aluminum foil tented over it.
4. Get the skillet or pan back up to heat. Add the port, shallot, blueberries, and the remaining salt and pepper to the pan. Scrape some browned pieces off the bottom of the skillet or pan with a wooden spoon. Reduce the heat to medium-low and bring to a simmer. Cook, stirring sometimes, and gently crushing the blueberries for around 4 minutes or until the liquid has reduced by half.
5. Whisk in the butter one slice at a time. Toss the meat back into the skillet or pan. Toss it once with the sauce to coat it. The rest of the sauce can be spooned over the meat before serving.

11.25 Ground Beef Chili with Tomatoes

Preparation time-10 minutes| Cook time-15 minutes| Total time-25 minutes| Servings-2|Difficulty-Easy

Nutritional Facts- Calories: 890; Total Fat: 20g; Total Carbs: 63g; Sugar: 13g; Fiber: 17g; Protein: 116g; Sodium: 562mg

Ingredients

- Half chopped onion
- One (14-ounce) can of kidney beans, drained
- Half pound of extra-lean ground beef
- One (28-ounce) can of chopped tomatoes, undrained
- Half tablespoon of chili powder
- A quarter teaspoon of sea salt
- Half teaspoon of garlic powder

Instructions

1. Cook the beef and onion in a big pot over medium-high heat for around 5 minutes, crumbling the beef with a wooden spoon until it browns.
2. Add the kidney beans, tomatoes, garlic powder, chili powder, salt, and stir to combine. Bring to a low boil, then reduce to low heat. Cook for 10 minutes, stirring occasionally.

11.26 Fish Taco Salad with Strawberry Avocado Salsa

Preparation time-20 minutes| Cook time-10 minutes| Total time-30 minutes| Servings-2|Difficulty-Easy

Nutritional Facts- Calories: 878; Total Fat: 26g; Total Carbs: 53g; Sugar: 15g; Fiber: 18g; Protein: 119g; Sodium: 582mg

Ingredients

For the salsa

- Two hulled and diced strawberries
- Half diced small shallot
- Two tablespoons of finely chopped fresh cilantro
- Two tablespoons of freshly squeezed lime juice
- 1/8 teaspoon of cayenne pepper
- Half diced avocado
- Two tablespoons of canned black beans, rinsed and drained
- One thinly sliced green onions
- Half teaspoon of finely chopped peeled ginger
- A quarter teaspoon of sea salt

For the fish

- One teaspoon of agave nectar
- Two cups of arugula
- One tablespoon of extra-virgin olive oil or avocado oil
- Half tablespoon of freshly squeezed lime juice
- One pound of light fish (halibut, cod, or red snapper), cut into two fillets
- A quarter teaspoon of freshly ground black pepper
- Half teaspoon of sea salt

Instructions

1. Preheat the grill, whether it's gas or charcoal.
2. To create the salsa, add the avocado, beans, strawberries, shallot, cilantro, green onions, salt, ginger, lime juice, and cayenne pepper in a medium mixing cup. Put aside after mixing until all of the components are well combined.
3. To render the salad, whisk together the agave, oil, and lime juice in a small bowl. Toss the arugula with the vinaigrette in a big mixing bowl.
4. Season the fish fillets with pepper and salt. Grill the fish for 7 to 9 minutes over direct high heat, flipping once during cooking. The fish should be translucent and quickly flake.

5. Place one cup of arugula salad on each plate to eat. Cover each salad with a fillet and a heaping spoonful of salsa.

11.27 Beef and Bell Pepper Stir-Fry

Preparation time-5 minutes| Cook time-10 minutes| Total time-15 minutes| Servings-2|Difficulty-Easy

Nutritional Facts- Calories: 599; Total Fat: 19g; Total Carbs: 9g; Sugar: 4g; Fiber: 2g; Protein: 97g; Sodium: 520mg

Ingredients

- Three scallions, white and green parts, chopped
- One tablespoon of grated fresh ginger
- Two minced garlic cloves
- Half pound of extra-lean ground beef
- One chopped red bell peppers
- A quarter teaspoon of sea salt

Instructions

1. Cook the beef for around 5 minutes in a big non-stick skillet or pan over medium-high heat, crumbling it with a wooden spoon until it browns.
2. Add the scallions, ginger, red bell peppers, and salt. Cook, sometimes stirring, for around 4 minutes or until the bell peppers are tender.
3. Garlic can be included now. Cook for 30 seconds while continuously stirring. Switch off the flame, and you are done.

11.28 Veggie Pizza with Cauliflower-Yam Crust

Preparation time-15 minutes| Cook time-0 minutes| Total time-15 minutes| Servings-2|Difficulty-Easy

Nutritional Facts- Calories: 4329; Total Fat: 17g; Total Carbs: 9g; Sugar: 3g; Fiber: 5g; Protein: 37g; Sodium: 430mg

Ingredients

- Half medium peeled and chopped garnet yam
- One teaspoon of sea salt, divided
- Half tablespoon of coconut oil, plus more for greasing pizza stone
- A quarter cup of sliced cremini mushrooms
- A quarter medium head cauliflower, broken into small florets
- Half tablespoon of dried Italian herbs
- Half cup flour of brown rice
- Half sliced small red onion
- Half zucchini or yellow summer squash

- Two tablespoons of vegan pesto
- Half cup of spinach

Instructions

1. Preheat the oven to 400 degrees Fahrenheit or preheat the pizza stone in case you have one.
2. In a big pot with 1 inch of water, place a steamer basket. Place the yam and cauliflower in the steamer basket and steam for 15 minutes, or until both are quickly pricked with a fork. If you overcook the vegetables, they can get too soggy.
3. Place the vegetables in a food blender or processor and process until smooth. Blend in the Italian herbs and half a teaspoon of salt until smooth. Place the mixture in a big mixing bowl. Gradually whisk in the flour until it is well mixed.
4. Use coconut oil to oil the pizza stone or a pizza plate. In the middle of the pizza stone, pile the cauliflower mixture. Spread the pizza dough uniformly in a round or circular fashion (much like frosting) with a spatula until the crust is around 1/8 inches thick. Bake for around 45 minutes. To get the top crispy, switch on the broiler and broil the crust for 2 minutes.
5. In a medium skillet or pan, melt the coconut oil over medium heat. Cook for 2 minutes after adding the onion. Add the squash, mushrooms, and the remaining ingredients to a large mixing bowl. Sauté for 3 to 4 minutes with a quarter teaspoon of salt. Remove the spinach from the heat as soon as it starts to wilt.
6. Evenly splatter the pesto around the pizza crust. Over the pesto, spread the sautéed vegetables. It's time to slice the pizza and eat it.

11.29 Toasted Pecan Quinoa Burgers

Preparation time-10 minutes| Cook time-30 minutes| Total time-40 minutes| Servings-2|Difficulty-Moderate

Nutritional Facts- Calories: 432; Total Fat: 12g; Total Carbs: 12g; Sugar: 5g; Fiber: 3g; Protein: 57g; Sodium: 566mg

Ingredients

- Two cups of vegetable broth, divided
- One teaspoon of sea salt, plus more for seasoning
- Two tablespoons of sesame seeds
- Half teaspoon of dried oregano
- A quarter cup of canned black beans, rinsed and drained
- Two tablespoons of pecans
- Half cup of quinoa, rinsed and drained
- A quarter cup of sunflower seeds
- Half teaspoon of ground cumin
- Half shredded carrot
- Freshly ground black pepper

- Half of the thinly sliced avocado
- Half teaspoon of coconut or sunflower oil

Instructions

1. Preheat oven to 375 degrees Fahrenheit.
2. Roast the pecans for 5 to 7 minutes on a baking sheet.
3. In a big saucepan, bring one cup of broth, quinoa, and salt to a boil over medium-high heat. Reduce the heat to a minimum, cover, and cook for 20 minutes, stirring occasionally.
4. In a food processor, grind the pecans, cumin, sesame seeds, sunflower seeds, and oregano to a medium-coarse texture.
5. Combine a half cup of quinoa, carrots, nut mixture, and beans in a big mixing bowl. Slowly pour the remaining cup of broth, constantly stirring, before the paste becomes tacky. Season with pepper and salt as per taste.
6. Form the mixture into two 1/2-inch-thick patties and cook, refrigerate them right away.
7. In a big skillet or pan over medium-high heat, melt the coconut oil. Cook for around 2 minutes on either side. Carry on for the remaining patty in the same manner. Avocado slices can be placed on top of the burgers.

11.30 Sizzling Salmon and Quinoa

Preparation time-10 minutes| Cook time-1 hour and 5 minutes| Total time-1 hour and 15 minutes| Servings-2|Difficulty-Easy

Nutritional Facts- Calories: 599; Total Fat: 20g; Total Carbs: 10g; Sugar: 4g; Fiber: 6g; Protein: 88g; Sodium: 662mg

Ingredients

- Half teaspoon of extra-virgin olive oil
- Half cup of quinoa, rinsed and drained
- A quarter-pound of sliced chanterelle mushrooms
- Half cup of frozen petite peas
- One tablespoon of chopped fresh basil
- One head of garlic
- One and a half cups of mushroom broth, divided
- One tablespoon of coconut oil
- Half cup of shredded brussels sprouts
- One tablespoon of nutritional yeast
- Half tablespoon of dried oregano
- Sea salt and freshly ground black pepper
- A quarter of a pound of salmon, skin, and bones removed, cut into 1-inch cubes

Instructions

1. Preheat oven to 350 degrees Fahrenheit.
2. Remove the top of the garlic head to reveal the cloves. Cover the head in foil and drizzle with olive oil. Place in the oven for 50 minutes to roast.
3. Meanwhile, in a big saucepan, mix one cup of broth and the quinoa. Bring to a boil over high heat, then reduce to low heat, cover, and simmer without stirring for 20 minutes. To make this dish, measure a quarter cup of quinoa, reserving any leftovers for another use.
4. Heat the coconut oil in a big skillet or pan over medium heat. Sauté for 5 minutes, or before the mushrooms release liquid and become tender. Sauté for 3 minutes with the brussels sprouts, adding up to a quarter cup of broth if required to keep the mushrooms and sprouts from sticking to the skillet or pan. Sauté for 5 minutes, stirring regularly, with the peas, basil, nutritional yeast, and oregano. Toss the salmon gently in the pan to mix. Squeeze the garlic cloves gently into the pan. Cook, covered, for 4 to 5 minutes, stirring periodically.
5. Stir in the remaining quarter cup of broth and quarter cup of quinoa in the skillet or pan until all is well mixed. Season with pepper and salt to taste and serve.

Chapter 12-Soups and Stews Recipes

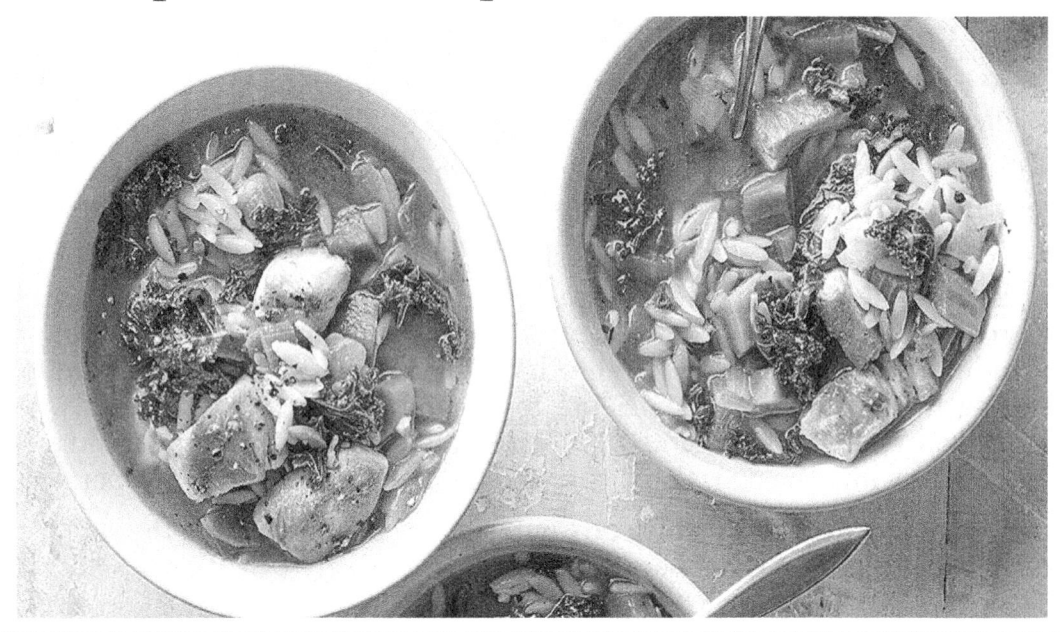

12.1 Roasted Vegetable Soup

Preparation time-30 minutes| Cook time-40 minutes| Total time-1 hour and 20 minutes| Servings-2|Difficulty-Hard

Nutritional Facts- Calories: 197; Total Fat: 17g; Total Carbohydrates: 13g; Sugar: 5g; Fiber: 3g; Protein: 2g; Sodium: 426mg

Ingredients

- A quarter head of cauliflower, broken into florets
- One halved shallot
- One garlic clove
- One teaspoon of salt
- One to three cups of water or vegetable broth
- One carrot halved lengthwise
- Half cup of cubed butternut squash
- One quartered Roma tomatoes
- Two tablespoons of extra-virgin olive oil
- 1/8 teaspoon of freshly ground black pepper

Instructions

1. Preheat the oven to 400 degrees Fahrenheit.
2. Combine the cauliflower, carrots, butternut squash, tomatoes, shallots, and garlic in a big mixing bowl. Toss the vegetables in salt, olive oil, and pepper to cover.
3. Arrange the veggies in a single layer on a rimmed baking sheet. Roast the vegetables for around 25 minutes, or until they begin to brown, on the sheet in the preheated oven.

4. In a big Dutch oven over high heat, move the roasted vegetables. Put to a boil with sufficient water to cover the vegetables. Reduce the heat to low heat and continue to steam the soup for another 10 minutes.

5. Pour the soup into a blender and puree until smooth, working in batches if necessary.

12.2 Broth Mushrooms

Preparation time-15 minutes| Cook time-10 minutes| Total time-25 minutes| Servings-2|Difficulty-Easy

Nutritional Facts- Calories: 111; Total Fat: 5g; Total Carbohydrates: 9g; Sugar: 4g; Fiber: 2g; Protein: 9g; Sodium: 1357mg

Ingredients

- One halved and thinly sliced onion
- Half finely chopped celery stalk
- Half teaspoon of salt
- Pinch of nutmeg
- One tablespoon of chopped fresh tarragon
- Half tablespoon of extra-virgin olive oil
- Two thinly sliced garlic cloves
- Half pound of thinly sliced mushrooms
- A quarter teaspoon of freshly ground black pepper
- Two cups of vegetable broth

Instructions

1. Heat the olive oil in a big pot over high heat.
2. Add the garlic, onion, and celery. Let it sauté for 3 minutes.
3. Add the mushrooms, pepper, salt, and nutmeg. Continue to sauté for another 5 to 10 minutes.
4. Bring the soup to a boil with the vegetable broth. Reduce the heat to a low setting and keep it there. Cook for a further 5 minutes.
5. Add the tarragon and serve.

12.3 Tomato Soup

Preparation time-10 minutes| Cook time-15 minutes| Total time-25 minutes| Servings-2|Difficulty-Easy

Nutritional Facts- Calories: 233; Total Fat: 7g; Total Carbs: 35g; Sugar: 24g; Fiber: 13g; Protein: 10g; Sodium: 577mg

Ingredients

- Half finely chopped onion
- One (28-ounce) can of crushed tomatoes, undrained

- One tablespoon of extra-virgin olive oil
- One minced garlic clove
- Two cups of no-salt-added vegetable broth
- 1/8 teaspoon of freshly ground black pepper
- Half teaspoon of sea salt

Instructions

1. Heat the olive oil in a big pot over medium-high heat until it starts shimmering.
2. Toss in the onion. Cook, stirring regularly, for around 7 minutes, or until browned.
3. Garlic can be included now. Cook for 30 seconds while continuously stirring.
4. Add the vegetable broth, tomatoes, pepper, and salt. Cook for 5 minutes on low heat.
5. Move the soup to a blender or an immersion blender with care. Blend until entirely smooth.

12.4 Cream of Kale Soup

Preparation time-10 minutes| Cook time-20 minutes| Total time-30 minutes| Servings-2|Difficulty-Easy

Nutritional Facts- Calories: 129; Total Fat: 7g; Total Carbs: 16g; Sugar: 6g; Fiber: 2g; Protein: 3g; Sodium: 302mg

Ingredients

- Half finely chopped onion
- Half cup of broccoli florets
- Half teaspoon of garlic powder
- 1/8 teaspoon of freshly ground black pepper
- Coconut milk (optional)
- One tablespoon of extra-virgin olive oil, plus extra for garnish, if desired
- Two cups of kale
- Three cups of no-salt vegetable broth
- Half teaspoon of sea salt
- Microgreens (optional)

Instructions

1. Heat the olive oil in a big pot over medium-high heat until it starts shimmering.
2. Cook, stirring regularly, for around 5 minutes, or until the onion is tender.
3. Add the broccoli, kale, garlic powder, vegetable broth, pepper, and salt. Bring to a simmer, then reduce to medium-low heat. Cook, occasionally stirring, for 10 to 15 minutes, or until the veggies are tender.
4. Blend until creamy, carefully transferring to a blender. Serve immediately with extra oil, coconut milk, and microgreens.

12.5 Squash and Ginger Soup

Preparation time-10 minutes| Cook time-20 minutes| Total time-30 minutes| Servings-2|Difficulty-Easy

Nutritional Facts- Calories: 96; Total Fat: 7g; Total Carbs: 9g; Sugar: 6g; Fiber: <1g; Protein: <1g; Sodium 266mg

Ingredients

- Half chopped onion
- Two minced garlic cloves
- One and a half cups of butternut squash (or acorn squash)
- 1/8 teaspoon of freshly ground black pepper
- Two tablespoons of microgreens
- One tablespoon of extra-virgin olive oil
- Half tablespoon of grated ginger
- Three cups of vegetable broth
- A quarter teaspoon of sea salt
- Two tablespoons of coconut milk

Instructions

1. Heat the olive oil in a big pot over medium-high heat until it starts shimmering.
2. Add the ginger and onion and cook, stirring regularly, for around 5 minutes, or until the onion is tender. Cook, stirring continuously, for another 30 seconds after adding the garlic.
3. Add the squash, vegetable broth, pepper, and salt. Cook for about 10 minutes, wrapped until the squash is tender.
4. Transfer to a blender with care. Blend until entirely smooth.
5. Serve with a dollop of coconut milk and microgreens.

12.6 Easy Summer Gazpacho

Preparation time-15 minutes| Cook time-0 minutes| Total time-15 minutes| Servings-2|Difficulty-Easy

Nutritional Facts- Calories: 165; Total Fat: 13g; Total Carbs: 12g; Sugar: 8g; Fiber: 3g; Protein: 3g; Sodium: 283mg

Ingredients

- Two tablespoons of extra-virgin olive oil
- One minced garlic clove
- Three chopped large heirloom tomatoes
- Two tablespoons of fresh basil leaves
- Juice of half a lemon

- Half to one teaspoon of hot sauce
- Zest of half a lemon

Instructions

1. Combine all of the ingredients in a blender.
2. For a chunkier soup, pulse 20 times in 1-second intervals, or blend until smooth for a more delicate texture.

12.7 Fennel, Leek, and Pear Soup

Preparation time-15 minutes| Cook time-15 minutes| Total time-30 minutes| Servings-2|Difficulty-Easy

Nutritional Facts- Calories: 267; Total Fat: 15g; Total Carbohydrates: 33g; Sugar: 13g; Fiber: 7g; Protein: 5g; Sodium: 627mg

Ingredients

- One sliced leek, white part only
- One pear, peeled, cored, and cut into 1/2-inch cubes
- 1/8 teaspoon of freshly ground black pepper
- One tablespoon of extra-virgin olive oil
- Half of a fennel bulb, cut into 1/4-inch-thick slices
- Half teaspoon of salt
- A quarter cup of cashews
- One cup of packed spinach or arugula
- One and a half cups of water or vegetable broth

Instructions

1. Heat the olive oil in a big Dutch oven over high heat.
2. Add the fennel and leeks. Let it sauté for 5 minutes.
3. Add the salt, pears, and pepper and continue to sauté for another 3 minutes.
4. Bring the soup to a boil with cashews and water. Reduce the heat to low and cook, partly covered, for 5 minutes.
5. Add the spinach and mix well.
6. Pour the soup into a blender and puree until creamy, operating in batches if possible.

12.8 Pumpkin Soup with Fried Sage

Preparation time-15 minutes| Cook time-10 minutes| Total time-25 minutes| Servings-3|Difficulty-Easy

Nutritional Facts- Calories: 379; Total Fat: 20g; Total Carbohydrates: 45g; Sugar: 17g; Fiber: 18g; Protein: 10g; Sodium: 1365mg

Ingredients

- Half chopped onion
- Half of one (15-ounce) can of pumpkin purée
- One teaspoon of chipotle powder
- A quarter teaspoon of freshly ground black pepper
- Six stemmed sage leaves
- Two tablespoons of extra-virgin olive oil
- One garlic clove, cut into 1/8-inch-thick slices
- Two cups of vegetable broth
- Half teaspoon of salt
- A quarter cup of vegetable oil

Instructions

1. Add the onion, olive oil, and garlic to a big, heavy Dutch over high heat. Cook for 5 minutes, or until the veggies are starting to brown.
2. Add the pumpkin, chipotle powder, vegetable broth, pepper, and salt. Get the liquid to a boil. Reduce the heat to low and continue to cook for another 5 minutes.
3. Place a medium sauté pan over high heat when the soup is simmering. Heat the vegetable oil until it is hot.
4. Toss each sage leaf gently into the oil and cook for 1 minute, or until crisp. Move the sage to paper towels to rinse using a slotted spoon. Remove the vegetable oil until it has cooled.
5. Pour the soup into bowls (if needed, puree the soup in a blender first), and top with three fried sage leaves per serving.

12.9 Lentil and Carrot Soup with Ginger

Preparation time-15 minutes| Cook time-10 minutes| Total time-25 minutes| Servings-2 |Difficulty-Easy

Nutritional Facts- Calories: 207; Total Fat: 5g; Total Carbohydrates: 28g; Sugar: 5g; Fiber: 10g; Protein: 14g; Sodium: 1430mg

Ingredients

- One thinly sliced carrot
- One peeled and thinly sliced garlic cloves
- One and a half cups of water or vegetable broth
- One tablespoon of chopped fresh cilantro, or parsley
- 1/8 teaspoon of freshly ground black pepper
- Half tablespoon of coconut oil
- Half small white onion, peeled and sliced thin

- Half tablespoon of chopped fresh ginger
- Half of one (15-ounce) can of lentils, drained and rinsed
- Half teaspoon of salt

Instructions

1. Melt the coconut oil in a big pot over medium-high flame. Add the carrots, garlic, onion, and ginger. Let it sauté for around five minutes.
2. Fill the pot halfway with water and bring it to a boil. Reduce the heat to low and cook, occasionally stirring, for around 5 minutes, or until the carrots are soft.
3. Add in the cilantro, lentils, pepper, and salt.
4. Stir and then serve.

12.10 Coconut Curry–Butternut Squash Soup

Preparation time-15 minutes| Cook time-4 hours| Total time-4 hours and 15 minutes| Servings-2|Difficulty-Hard

Nutritional Facts- Calories: 416; Total Fat: 31g; Total Carbohydrates: 30g; Sugar: 13g; Fiber: 7g; Protein: 10g; Sodium: 1387mg

Ingredients

- Half a pound of butternut squash, peeled and cut into 1-inch cubes
- Half sliced onion
- A quarter cup of no-added-sugar apple juice
- Half of one (13.5-ounce) can of coconut milk
- One tablespoon of coconut oil
- Half of one small head of cauliflower, cut into 1-inch pieces
- Half tablespoon of curry powder
- Two cups of vegetable broth
- Half teaspoon of salt
- Two tablespoons of chopped fresh cilantro, divided
- 1/8 teaspoon of freshly ground white pepper

Instructions

1. Add the butternut squash, onion, cauliflower, curry powder, vegetable broth, apple juice, coconut milk, cinnamon, and white pepper in a slow cooker. Set the timer for 4 hours on heavy.
2. Serve the soup as is or mix it to a smooth consistency before eating.
3. Serve with cilantro as a garnish.

12.11 Soba Noodle Soup with Spinach

Preparation time-15 minutes| Cook time-10 minutes| Total time-25 minutes| Servings-2|Difficulty-Easy

Nutritional Facts- Calories: 255; Total Fat: 9g; Total Carbohydrates: 34g; Sugar: 4g; Fiber: 4g; Protein: 13g; Sodium: 1774mg

Ingredients

- Four ounces of shiitake mushrooms stemmed and sliced thin
- One minced garlic clove
- Half teaspoon of salt
- One and a half cups of water
- One tablespoon of coconut oil
- Two thinly sliced scallions
- Half tablespoon of minced fresh ginger
- Two cups of vegetable broth
- Two ounces of buckwheat soba noodles
- Half tablespoon of freshly squeezed lemon juice
- Half a bunch of spinach washed and cut into strips

Instructions

1. Heat the coconut oil in a big pot over low heat.
2. Add the mushrooms, ginger, garlic, scallions, and salt to a large mixing bowl. Let it sauté for around five minutes.
3. Get the vegetable broth and water to a boil in the pot. Cook for 5 minutes after adding the soba noodles.
4. Turn off the heat in the pot. Add in the spinach and lemon juice. Serve it hot immediately.

12.12 Sweet Potato and Rice Soup

Preparation time-15 minutes| Cook time-15 minutes| Total time-30 minutes| Servings-2 |Difficulty-Easy

Nutritional Facts- Calories: 167; Total Fat: 2g; Total Carbohydrates: 29g; Sugar: 7g; Fiber: 3g; Protein: 8g; Sodium: 789mg

Ingredients

- One medium sweet potato, peeled and cut into 1-inch cubes
- One thinly sliced garlic clove
- Half bunch of broccolini, cut into 1-inch pieces
- Two tablespoons of fresh cilantro leaves
- Two cups of vegetable broth

- One coarsely chopped onion
- One teaspoon of minced fresh ginger
- Half cup of cooked basmati rice

Instructions

1. Bring the broth to a boil in a big Dutch oven over high flame.
2. Add the onion, sweet potato, ginger, and garlic. Cook, sometimes stirring, for 5 to 8 minutes, or until the sweet potato is tender.
3. Simmer for a further 3 minutes after adding the broccolini.
4. Turn off the heat. Mix in the rice and cilantro.

12.13 Broccoli and Lentil Stew

Preparation time-15 minutes| Cook time-30 minutes| Total time-45 minutes| Servings-2|Difficulty-Moderate

Nutritional Facts- Calories: 182; Total Fat: 6g; Total Carbohydrates: 24g; Sugar: 5g; Fiber: 9g; Protein: 11g; Sodium: 1233mg

Ingredients

- Half of one small finely chopped onion
- One minced clove of garlic
- Half cup of dried green or brown lentils
- Three cups of broccoli florets
- 1/8 teaspoon of freshly ground black pepper
- Two tablespoons of chopped fresh Italian parsley
- Half tablespoon of extra-virgin olive oil, plus additional for drizzling
- Half small chopped carrot
- One cup of vegetable broth
- Half teaspoon of dried oregano
- Half teaspoon of salt
- A quarter cup of sliced pitted green olives

Instructions

1. Heat the olive oil in a big pot over high heat.
2. Add the carrot, onion, and garlic and sauté it for around five minutes.
3. Add and bring the lentils, vegetable broth, and oregano to a boil. Reduce the heat to a low. Cook the lentils in the soup for 15 to 20 minutes or until they are soft.
4. Cover the pot and continue to cook for another 5 minutes.
5. Stir in the parsley and olives after removing the pot from the heat. Stir in any water if the soup is too thick.

6. Pour the soup into the bowls and top with a drizzle of olive oil before serving.

12.14 Winter Squash and Kasha Stew

Preparation time-15 minutes| Cook time-4 hours| Total time-4 hours and 15 minutes| Servings-2|Difficulty-Hard

Nutritional Facts- Calories: 325; Total Fat: 6g; Total Carbohydrates: 60g; Sugar: 2g; Fiber: 8g; Protein: 12g; Sodium: 1231mg

Ingredients

- One pound of peeled and cubed winter squash
- One thinly sliced leek, white part only
- Half cup of rinsed kasha
- A quarter teaspoon of freshly ground black pepper
- Two cups of thoroughly washed and stemmed chopped kale
- Half tablespoon of extra-virgin olive oil
- Half of one thinly sliced fennel bulb
- One chopped garlic clove
- Half teaspoon of salt
- One and a half cups of water or vegetable broth

Instructions

1. Add the squash, olive oil, fennel, garlic, leeks, kasha, pepper, salt, and water in a slow cooker.
2. Set the timer for 4 hours on high.
3. Stir in the kale just before eating. The stew's heat can cause it to wilt, making it easier to chew and digest.

12.15 Chicken Chili with Beans

Preparation time-15 minutes| Cook time-4 hours| Total time-4 hours and 15 minutes| Servings-2|Difficulty-Hard

Nutritional Facts- Calories: 423; Total Fat: 13g; Total Carbohydrates: 41g; Sugar: 6g; Fiber: 10g; Protein: 42g; Sodium: 857mg

Ingredients

- One chopped onion
- One chopped celery stalk
- One teaspoon of salt
- Half teaspoon of freshly ground black pepper
- One teaspoon of dried oregano
- Half of one (28-ounce) can of chopped tomatoes
- One tablespoon of extra-virgin olive oil

- Two minced garlic cloves
- One teaspoon of ground cumin
- One teaspoon of chipotle powder
- Two boneless skinless chicken breasts, cut into 1-inch pieces
- One bay leaf
- Two cups of chicken broth, plus additional as needed
- Two tablespoons of chopped fresh parsley, divided
- One (15-ounce) can of white beans, drained and rinsed

Instructions

1. Add the onions, olive oil, garlic, cumin, celery, salt, pepper, chipotle powder, chicken, bay leaf, oregano, chicken broth, tomatoes, and white beans to the slow cooker.
2. Set the heat to high and cook it for 4 hours.
3. If the sauce becomes too deep, thin it out with a little more chicken broth or water.
4. Sprinkle parsley on top of each serving. Serve on its own or with brown rice or quinoa.

12.16 Mango and Black Bean Stew

Preparation time-10 minutes| Cook time-10 minutes| Total time-20 minutes| Servings-2|Difficulty-Easy

Nutritional Facts- Calories: 431; Total Fat: 9g; Total Carbohydrates: 72g; Sugar: 17g; Fiber: 22g; Protein: 20g; Sodium: 609mg

Ingredients

- Half chopped onion
- Half tablespoon of chili powder
- A quarter teaspoon of freshly ground black pepper
- One thinly sliced ripe mangos
- A quarter cup of sliced scallions
- One tablespoon of coconut oil
- One (15-ounce) can of black beans, drained and rinsed
- One teaspoon of salt
- Half cup of water
- Two tablespoons of chopped fresh cilantro

Instructions

1. Melt the coconut oil in a big pot over a high flame.
2. Cook for 5 minutes after adding the onion.
3. Combine the black beans, pepper, chili powder, salt, and water in a large mixing bowl. Get the water to a simmer. Reduce the heat to low and continue to cook for another 5 minutes.

4. Remove the pot from the heat, and just before eating, mix in the mangos. Serve with cilantro and scallions on the side.

12.17 Coconut Fish Stew

Preparation time-15 minutes| Cook time-10 minutes| Total time-25 minutes| Servings-2|Difficulty-Easy

Nutritional Facts- Calories: 608; Total Fat: 43g; Total Carbohydrates: 13g; Sugar: 7g; Fiber: 4g; Protein: 46g; Sodium: 725mg

Ingredients

- One thinly sliced white onion
- One thinly sliced zucchini
- One 4-inch piece lemongrass (white part only), bruised with the back of a knife
- One teaspoon of salt
- A quarter cup of slivered scallions
- Two tablespoons of freshly squeezed lemon juice
- Two tablespoons of coconut oil
- Two thinly sliced garlic cloves
- One pound of firm white fish fillet, cut into 1-inch cubes
- Half of one (13.5-ounce) can of coconut milk
- A quarter teaspoon of freshly ground white pepper
- Two tablespoons of chopped cilantro

Instructions

1. Melt the coconut oil in a big pot over medium heat.
2. Add the garlic, onion, and zucchini to a mixing bowl. For around 5 minutes, sauté it.
3. In a large pot, combine the fish, salt, coconut milk, lemongrass, and white pepper. If the liquid isn't enough to cover the fish, add more water. Bring to a boil, then reduce to low heat and continue cooking for 5 minutes.
4. Add the cilantro, scallions, and lemon juice to the soup as a garnish.

12.18 Gingered Chicken and Vegetable Soup

Preparation time-10 minutes| Cook time-10 minutes| Total time-20 minutes| Servings-2|Difficulty-Easy

Nutritional Facts- Calories: 341; Total Fat: 15g; Total Carbs: 11g; Sugar: 8g; Fiber: 1g; Protein: 40g; Sodium: 577mg

Ingredients

- Half chopped onion
- One tablespoon of grated fresh ginger

- Four cups no-salt-added chicken broth
- 1/8 teaspoon of freshly ground black pepper
- Two tablespoons of extra-virgin olive oil
- One chopped red bell pepper
- One and a half of shredded rotisserie chicken, skin removed
- Half teaspoon of sea salt

Instructions

1. Heat the olive oil in a big pot over medium-high heat until it starts shimmering.
2. Add the red bell peppers, onion, and ginger. Cook, stirring regularly, for around 5 minutes, or until the vegetables are tender.
3. Add the chicken, salt, chicken broth, and pepper. Bring to a low boil, then reduce to low heat. Reduce the heat to medium-low and continue to cook for another 5 minutes.

12.19 Curried Sweet Potato Soup

Preparation time-10 minutes| Cook time-15 minutes| Total time-25 minutes| Servings-2|Difficulty-Easy

Nutritional Facts- Calories: 253; Total Fat: 7g; Total Carbs: 45g; Sugar: 2g; Fiber: 7g; Protein: 3g; Sodium: 261mg

Ingredients

- Half chopped onion
- Four cups of no-salt-added vegetable broth
- Half teaspoon of ground turmeric
- 1/8 teaspoon of freshly ground black pepper
- Two tablespoons of extra-virgin olive oil
- Two cups of cubed, peeled sweet potato
- One teaspoon of curry powder
- Half teaspoon of sea salt

Instructions

1. Heat the olive oil in a big pot over medium-high heat until it starts shimmering.
2. Toss in the onion. Cook, stirring regularly, for around 5 minutes, or until tender.
3. Add the vegetable broth, sweet potato, curry powder, salt, turmeric, and pepper. Get the water to a simmer. Reduce the heat to medium-low and cook the sweet potato cubes for around 10 minutes or until they are tender.
4. Blend until creamy after transferring it to a blender.

12.20 Melon and Green Tea Soup

Preparation time-5 minutes| Cook time-0 minutes| Total time-5 minutes| Servings-2|Difficulty-Easy

Nutritional Facts- Calories: 168; Total Fat: <1g; Total Carbs: 40g; Sugar: 36g; Fiber: 3g; Protein: 5g; Sodium: 73mg

Ingredients

- One cup of cubed honeydew melon
- One tablespoon of honey
- A quarter cup of non-fat Greek yogurt
- One tablespoon of matcha
- One tablespoon of chopped fresh mint, plus more for garnish
- A quarter cup of water

Instructions

1. In a blender or food processor, combine the matcha, melon, mint, honey, water, and yogurt.
2. Blend until smooth. Garnish with mint sprigs.

12.21 Beefy Lentil and Tomato Stew

Preparation time-10 minutes| Cook time-10 minutes| Total time-20 minutes| Servings-2|Difficulty-Easy

Nutritional Facts- Calories: 461; Total Fat: 15g; Total Carbs: 37g; Sugar: 2g; Fiber: 17g; Protein: 44g; Sodium: 321mg

Ingredients

- Half a pound of extra-lean ground beef
- Half of one (14-ounce) can of lentils, drained
- Two tablespoons of extra-virgin olive oil
- Half chopped onion
- Half of one (14-ounce) can of chopped tomatoes with garlic and basil, drained
- 1/8 teaspoon of freshly ground black pepper
- Half teaspoon of sea salt

Instructions

1. Heat the olive oil in a big pot over medium-high heat until it starts shimmering.
2. Add the onion and beef. Cook, crumbling the beef with a wooden spoon until it browns, around 5 minutes.
3. Add the lentils, salt, tomatoes, and pepper. Bring to a low boil, then reduce to low heat. Turn the heat down to medium. Cook, occasionally stirring, for 3 to 4 minutes, or until the lentils are warm.

12.22 Garlicky Lamb Stew

Preparation time-15 minutes| Cook time-15 minutes| Total time-30 minutes| Servings-2|Difficulty-Easy

Nutritional Facts- Calories: 295; Total Fat: 12g; Total Carbs: 12g; Sugar: 7g; Fiber: 3g; Protein: 34g; Sodium: 332mg

Ingredients

- One tablespoon of extra-virgin olive oil
- One teaspoon of dried oregano
- A quarter teaspoon of freshly ground black pepper
- Three minced garlic cloves
- Half a pound of ground lamb
- Half chopped onion
- Half teaspoon of sea salt
- Half of one (28-ounce) can of chopped tomatoes, drained

Instructions

1. Cook the lamb for around 5 minutes in a big non-stick skillet or pan over medium-high heat, crumbling it with a wooden spoon until it browns. Drain the fat and transfer the lamb to a serving platter.
2. Return the skillet or pan to heat and drizzle in the olive oil until it shimmers.
3. Add the onion, salt, oregano, and pepper. Cook, sometimes stirring, for 5 minutes, or until the onions are tender.
4. Return the lamb to the skillet or pan with the tomatoes and stir to combine. Cook for 3 minutes, or until well cooked, stirring periodically.
5. Garlic can be included now. Cook for 30 seconds while continuously stirring.

Chapter 13-Sides and salads Recipes

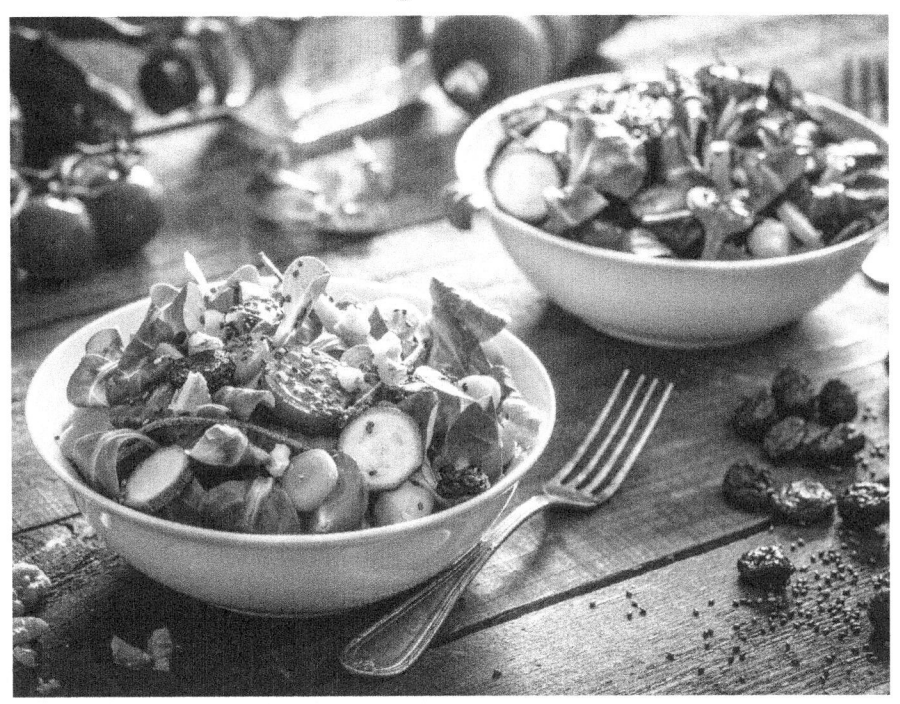

13.1 Broccoli-Sesame Stir-Fry

Preparation time-10 minutes| Cook time-8 minutes| Total time-18 minutes| Servings-2|Difficulty-Easy

Nutritional Facts- Calories: 134; Total Fat: 11g; Total Carbs: 9g; Sugar: 2g; Fiber: 3g; Protein: 4g; Sodium: 148mg

Ingredients

- One teaspoon of sesame oil
- One tablespoon of grated fresh ginger
- Two tablespoons of extra-virgin olive oil
- Two cups of broccoli florets
- 1/8 teaspoon of sea salt
- One tablespoon of toasted sesame seeds
- Two minced garlic cloves

Instructions

1. Heat the olive oil and sesame oil in a big nonstick skillet or pan over medium-high heat until they shimmer.
2. Add the ginger, broccoli, and salt. Cook, constantly stirring, for 5 to 7 minutes, or until the broccoli starts to brown.
3. Garlic can be included now. Cook for 30 seconds while continuously stirring.
4. Remove the skillet or pan from the heat and add the sesame seeds.

13.2 Salmon and Dill Pâté

Preparation time-10 minutes| Cook time-0 minutes| Total time-10 minutes| Servings-2|Difficulty-Easy

Nutritional Facts- Calories: 197; Total Fat: 11g; Total Carbs: <1g; Sugar: 0g; Fiber: <1g; Protein: 25g; Sodium: 295mg

Ingredients

- Two tablespoons of heavy (whipping) cream
- Three ounces of cooked salmon, bones, and skin removed
- One tablespoon of chopped fresh dill or 1½two teaspoons of dried
- Half teaspoon of sea salt
- Zest of one lemon

Instructions

1. In a blender or food processor (or in a large bowl using a mixer), combine the salmon, heavy cream, dill, lemon zest, and salt.
2. Blend until smooth.

13.3 Chickpea and Garlic Hummus

Preparation time-5 minutes| Cook time-0 minutes| Total time-5 minutes| Servings-2|Difficulty-Easy

Nutritional Facts- Calories: 178; Total Fat: 9g; Total Carbs: 19g; Sugar: 3g; Fiber: 6g; Protein: 7g; Sodium: 171mg

Ingredients

- Two tablespoons of extra-virgin olive oil (plus extra for garnish, if desired)
- Half of one (14-ounce) can chickpeas, drained
- Two minced garlic cloves
- One tablespoon of tahini
- Juice of one lemon
- Paprika, for garnish (optional)
- Half teaspoon of sea salt

Instructions

1. In a blender or food processor, combine all the ingredients. Blend until smooth.
2. Garnish as desired.

13.4 Citrus Spinach

Preparation time-10 minutes| Cook time-7 minutes| Total time-17 minutes| Servings-2|Difficulty-Easy

Nutritional Facts- Calories: 80; Total Fat: 7g; Total Carbs: 4g; Sugar: 2g; Fiber: 1g; Protein: 1g; Sodium: 258mg

Ingredients

- Two cups of fresh baby spinach
- Juice of half orange
- One tablespoon of extra-virgin olive oil
- Two minced garlic cloves
- Zest of half orange
- 1/8 teaspoon of freshly ground black pepper
- Half teaspoon of sea salt

Instructions

1. Heat the olive oil in a big skillet or pan over medium-high heat until it starts shimmering.
2. Cook, stirring regularly, for 3 minutes after adding the spinach.
3. Garlic can be included now. Cook for 30 seconds while continuously stirring.
4. Add the orange zest, orange juice, pepper, and salt. Cook, stirring continuously, for around 2 minutes, or until the juice has evaporated.

13.5 Brown Rice with Bell Peppers

Preparation time-10 minutes| Cook time-10 minutes| Total time-20 minutes| Servings-2|Difficulty-Easy

Nutritional Facts- Calories: 266; Total Fat: 8g; Total Carbs: 44g; Sugar: 4g; Fiber: 3g; Protein: 5g; Sodium: 455mg

Ingredients

- One chopped red bell pepper
- Half chopped onion
- One tablespoon of low-sodium soy sauce
- One tablespoon of extra-virgin olive oil
- Half chopped green bell pepper
- One cup of cooked brown rice

Instructions

1. Heat the olive oil in a big nonstick skillet or pan over medium-high heat until it starts shimmering.

2. Add the red and green bell peppers, as well as the onion. Cook, stirring regularly, for around 7 minutes, or until the veggies begin to brown.
3. Add the rice and soy sauce. Cook, stirring continuously, for around 3 minutes, or until the rice is warmed through.

13.6 Guacamole

Preparation time-10 minutes| Cook time-0 minutes| Total time-10 minutes| Servings-2|Difficulty-Easy

Nutritional Facts- Calories: 215; Total Fat: 20g; Total Carbs: 11g; Sugar: 1g; Fiber: 7g; Protein: 2g; Sodium: 243mg

Ingredients

- Half minced red onion
- Juice of one lime
- Half teaspoon of sea salt
- One peeled pitted and cubed avocado
- Two finely minced garlic cloves
- One tablespoon of chopped fresh cilantro leaves

Instructions

1. Mix the red onion, avocados, garlic, cilantro, lime juice, and salt in a medium mixing bowl.
2. To combine, lightly mash with a fork, and you are done.

13.7 Spinach and Walnut Salad with Raspberry Vinaigrette

Preparation time-10 minutes| Cook time-0 minutes| Total time-10 minutes| Servings-2|Difficulty-Easy

Nutritional Facts- Calories: 501; Total Fat: 50g; Total Carbs: 9g; Sugar: 2g; Fiber: 5g; Protein: 11g; Sodium: 96mg

Ingredients

- Two cups fresh baby spinach
- Two tablespoons of raspberry vinaigrette
- Two tablespoons of walnut pieces

Instructions

1. Combine the walnuts and spinach in a medium mixing bowl.
2. Toss it with the vinaigrette and serve right away.

13.8 Tomato and Basil Salad

Preparation time-10 minutes| Cook time-0 minutes| Total time-10 minutes| Servings-2|Difficulty-Easy

Nutritional Facts- Calories: 140; Total Fat: 14g; Total Carbs: 4g; Sugar: 3g; Fiber: 1g; Protein: 1g; Sodium: 239mg

Ingredients

- A quarter cup of fresh basil leaves, torn
- A quarter cup of extra-virgin olive oil
- A quarter teaspoon of freshly ground black pepper
- Four chopped large heirloom tomatoes
- Two finely minced garlic cloves
- Half teaspoon of sea salt

Instructions

1. Gently combine the tomatoes, garlic, basil, olive oil, pepper, and salt in a medium mixing bowl, and you are done.

13.9 Sautéed Apples and Ginger

Preparation time-10 minutes| Cook time-10 minutes| Total time-20 minutes| Servings-2|Difficulty-Easy

Nutritional Facts- Calories: 152; Total Fat: 7g; Total Carbs: 24g; Sugar: 18g; Fiber: 5g; Protein: <1g; Sodium: 60mg

Ingredients

- One and a half-peeled, cored, and sliced apple
- One teaspoon of ground cinnamon
- Pinch of sea salt
- One tablespoon of coconut oil
- Half tablespoon of grated fresh ginger
- A half packet of stevia

Instructions

1. Heat the coconut oil in a big nonstick skillet or pan over medium-high heat until it starts shimmering.
2. Add the apples, stevia, cinnamon, ginger, and salt. Cook, stirring regularly, for 7 to 10 minutes, or until the apples are tender.

13.10 Rosemary and Garlic Sweet Potatoes

Preparation time-10 minutes| Cook time-15 minutes| Total time-25 minutes| Servings-2|Difficulty-Easy

Nutritional Facts- Calories: 199; Total Fat: 7g; Total Carbs: 33g; Sugar: <1g; Fiber: 5g; Protein: 2g; Sodium: 245mg

Ingredients

- One sweet potato (skin left on), cut into 1/2-inch cubes
- Half teaspoon of sea salt

- Two tablespoons of freshly ground black pepper
- One tablespoon of extra-virgin olive oil
- Half tablespoon of chopped fresh rosemary leaves
- Two minced garlic cloves

Instructions

1. Heat the olive oil in a big nonstick skillet or pan over medium-high heat until it starts shimmering.
2. Add the rosemary, sweet potatoes, and salt. Cook, stirring regularly, for 10 to 15 minutes, or until the sweet potatoes begin to tan.
3. Garlic and pepper can be included now. Cook for 30 seconds while continuously stirring.

13.11 Mixed Berry Salad with Ginger

Preparation time-10 minutes| Cook time-0 minutes| Total time-10 minutes| Servings-2|Difficulty-Easy

Nutritional Facts- Calories: 75; Total Fat: <1g; Total Carbs: 18g; Sugar: 11g; Fiber: 5g; Protein: 1g; Sodium: 1mg

Ingredients

- Half cup of fresh raspberries
- Half tablespoon of grated fresh ginger
- Juice of one orange
- Half cup of fresh blueberries
- Half cup of fresh strawberries
- Zest of half orange

Instructions

1. In a medium bowl, stir together the raspberries, blueberries, strawberries, orange zest, ginger, and orange juice to mix well.

13.12 Pear-Walnut Salad

Preparation time-10 minutes| Cook time-0 minutes| Total time-10 minutes| Servings-2|Difficulty-Easy

Nutritional Facts- Calories: 263; Total Fat: 12g; Total Carbs: 41g; Sugar: 29g; Fiber: 7g; Protein: 3g; Sodium: 3mg

Ingredients

- Two tablespoons of chopped walnuts
- Two pears, peeled, cored, and chopped
- One tablespoon of honey
- One tablespoon of extra-virgin olive oil

- One tablespoon of balsamic vinegar

Instructions

1. Combine the walnuts and pears in a medium mixing bowl.
2. Whisk together balsamic vinegar, honey, and olive oil in a small bowl.
3. Pour the vinegar liquid over walnuts and pears and toss it a little, and you are done.

13.13 Sliced Apple, Beet, and Celery Salad

Preparation time-15 minutes| Cook time-0 minutes| Total time-15 minutes| Servings-2|Difficulty-Easy

Nutritional Facts- Calories: 239; Total Fat: 15g; Total Carbohydrates: 27g; Sugar: 18g; Fiber: 5g; Protein: 4g; Sodium: 121mg

Ingredients

- One small peeled and quartered beet
- One thinly sliced celery stalk
- A quarter cup of shredded carrots
- Half tablespoon of raw honey or maple syrup
- Salt as per taste
- Two tablespoons of pumpkin seeds
- One green cored and quartered apple
- Two cups of spinach
- Half thinly sliced red onion
- Half tablespoon of apple cider vinegar
- One and a half tablespoons of extra-virgin olive oil
- Freshly ground black pepper

Instructions

1. Slice the apples and beets with a meat slicer or the cutting disc of a food processor.
2. On a big platter, spread out the spinach. Over the spinach, arrange the beet and apples. Add the red onion, celery, and carrots on top.
3. Whisk together the honey, cider vinegar, pepper, salt, and olive oil in a shallow bowl.
4. Drizzle the dressing on top of the salad and sprinkle the pumpkin seeds on top.

13.14 Avocado and Mango Salad

Preparation time-15 minutes| Cook time-0 minutes| Total time-15 minutes| Servings-2|Difficulty-Easy

Nutritional Facts- Calories: 253; Total Fat: 13g; Total Carbohydrates: 37g; Sugar: 21g; Fiber: 10g; Protein: 4g; Sodium: 363mg

Ingredients

- Half cucumber, peeled, and cut into ¼-inch cubes
- One thinly sliced scallion
- Half cup of Creamy Coconut-Herb Dressing
- One chopped romaine lettuce hearts
- One ripe mango, cut into ½-inch cubes
- Half large ripe avocado

Instructions

1. Combine the cucumber, scallions, romaine lettuce, mangos, and avocado in a big serving bowl.
2. Dress the fruit and vegetables with the Creamy Coconut-Herb Dressing. Toss everything together.

13.15 Almost Caesar Salad

Preparation time-15 minutes| Cook time-0 minutes| Total time-15 minutes| Servings-2|Difficulty-Easy

Nutritional Facts- Calories: 431; Total Fat: 42g; Total Carbohydrates: 14g; Sugar: 3g; Fiber: 5g; Protein: 6g; Sodium: 803mg

Ingredients

- Half of one (14-ounce) can heart of palm, drained and sliced
- Half cup of almost Caesar Dressing
- Freshly ground black pepper
- One chopped romaine lettuce hearts
- A quarter cup of sunflower seeds
- Salt

Instructions

1. Combine the hearts of palm, romaine lettuce, and sunflower seeds in a big mixing bowl.
2. Toss the lettuce leaves with just enough dressing to gently cover them. Save the leftover dressing for another day.
3. Serve the salad after seasoning it with a pinch of pepper and salt.

13.16 Brussels Sprout Slaw

Preparation time-15 minutes| Cook time-0 minutes| Total time-15 minutes| Servings-2|Difficulty-Easy

Nutritional Facts- Calories: 189; Total Fat: 8g; Total Carbohydrates: 29g; Sugar: 13g; Fiber: 9g; Protein: 6g; Sodium: 678mg

Ingredients

- Half thinly sliced red onion

- Half teaspoon of Dijon mustard
- Half tablespoon of raw honey or maple syrup
- Half cup of plain coconut milk yogurt
- A quarter cup of pomegranate seeds
- Half pound of Brussels sprouts, stem ends removed and sliced thin
- Half cored and thinly sliced apple
- Half teaspoon of salt
- One teaspoon of apple cider vinegar
- A quarter cup of chopped toasted hazelnuts

Instructions

1. Combine the onion, brussels sprouts, and apple in a medium mixing dish.
2. Whisk together the cider vinegar, salt, Dijon mustard, honey, and yogurt in a shallow bowl.
3. Toss the Brussels sprouts with the dressing, so they are finely covered.
4. Arrange the pomegranate seeds and hazelnuts on top of the salad.

13.17 Vegetable Slaw with Feta Cheese

Preparation time-20 minutes| Cook time-0 minutes| Total time-20 minutes| Servings-2|Difficulty-Easy

Nutritional Facts- Calories: 388; Total Fat: 30g; Total Carbohydrates: 26g; Sugar: 12g; Fiber: 6g; Protein: 8g; Sodium: 981mg

Ingredients

- A quarter cup of apple cider vinegar
- Half teaspoon of Dijon mustard
- 1/8 teaspoon of freshly ground black pepper
- One peeled and shredded carrots
- Half peeled and shredded large beet
- Half thinly sliced small red onion
- One and a half ounces of crumbled feta cheese
- A quarter cup of extra-virgin olive oil
- Half tablespoon of raw honey or maple syrup
- Half teaspoon of salt
- One peeled and shredded large broccoli stem
- A quarter peeled and shredded celery root bulb
- One shredded zucchini
- One tablespoon of chopped fresh Italian parsley

Instructions

1. Whisk together the cider vinegar, olive oil, honey, salt, Dijon mustard, and pepper in a big mixing bowl.
2. Broccoli, celery root, carrots, beets, onion, zucchini, and Italian parsley can all be added at this stage. Toss the vegetables in the dressing to cover them.
3. Serve the slaw in a serving bowl with the feta cheese on top.

13.18 Mediterranean Chopped Salad

Preparation time-15 minutes| Cook time-0 minutes| Total time-15 minutes| Servings-2|Difficulty-Easy

Nutritional Facts- Calories: 194; Total Fat: 14g; Total Carbohydrates: 15g; Sugar: 7g; Fiber: 5g; Protein: 4g; Sodium: 661mg

Ingredients

- Two diced large tomatoes
- Half peeled and diced English cucumber
- One minced garlic clove
- Half tablespoon of chopped fresh parsley
- Two tablespoons of extra-virgin olive oil
- Half tablespoon of apple cider vinegar
- One cup of packed spinach
- Half thinly sliced bunch of radishes
- Half sliced scallion
- Half tablespoon of chopped fresh mint
- Half cup of unsweetened plain almond yogurt
- One and a half tablespoons of freshly squeezed lemon juice
- Half teaspoon of salt
- Half tablespoon of sumac
- 1/8 teaspoon of freshly ground black pepper

Instructions

1. Combine the spinach, radishes, tomatoes, cucumber, garlic, scallions, mint, parsley, yogurt, lemon juice, olive oil, cider vinegar, pepper, salt, and sumac together in a wide mixing bowl. Toss all around.

13.19 Quinoa and Roasted Asparagus Salad

Preparation time-10 minutes| Cook time-15 minutes| Total time-15 minutes| Servings-2|Difficulty-Easy

Nutritional Facts- Calories: 228; Total Fat: 13g; Total Carbohydrates: 24g; Sugar: 2g; Fiber: 5g; Protein: 6g; Sodium: 592mg

Ingredients

- One and a half tablespoons of extra-virgin olive oil
- One cup of cooked quinoa, cold or at room temperature
- Half tablespoon of apple cider vinegar
- Half bunch of trimmed asparagus
- One teaspoon of salt, plus additional for seasoning
- A quarter of a finely chopped red onion
- Two tablespoons of chopped fresh mint
- Freshly ground black pepper as per taste
- Half tablespoon of flaxseed

Instructions

1. Preheat the oven to 400 degrees Fahrenheit.
2. Mix the asparagus with half of salt and olive oil in a big mixing bowl.
3. Wrap the asparagus in a single layer of aluminum foil and put it on a baking sheet. Roast the asparagus for 10 to 15 minutes on a baking sheet in a preheated oven.
4. In a big mixing bowl, blend the onion, quinoa, vinegar, flaxseed, mint, and the remaining olive oil by the time the asparagus is roasting.
5. Cut the asparagus into 1/2-inch sections until it has cooled enough to treat. Season with pepper and salt before adding to the quinoa.

13.20 White Bean and Tuna Salad

Preparation time-15 minutes| Cook time-0 minutes| Total time-15 minutes| Servings-2|Difficulty-Easy

Nutritional Facts- Calories: 373; Total Fat: 19g; Total Carbohydrates: 28g; Sugar: 3g; Fiber: 7g; Protein: 29g; Sodium: 388mg

Ingredients

- One (5-ounce) can of flaked white tuna, drained
- A half-pint of cherry tomatoes halved lengthwise
- A quarter cup of pitted Kalamata olives
- One tablespoon of freshly squeezed lemon juice
- Two cups of arugula
- Half of one (15-ounce) can of white beans, drained and rinsed
- Half finely chopped red onion
- Two tablespoons of extra-virgin olive oil
- Salt as per taste
- One ounce of crumbled sheep's milk or goat's milk feta cheese

- Freshly ground black pepper as per taste

Instructions

1. Combine the arugula, white beans, tuna, olive oil, tomatoes, olives, onion, and lemon juice in a big mixing bowl. Add pepper and salt as per taste.
2. Serve the salad with feta cheese on top only before serving.

13.21 Mango Salsa

Preparation time-15 minutes| Cook time-0 minutes| Total time-15 minutes| Servings-One cup |Difficulty-Easy

Nutritional Facts- Calories: 40; Total Fat: 0g; Total Carbohydrates: 10g; Sugar: 8g; Fiber: 1g; Protein: 0g; Sodium: 98mg

Ingredients

- Half cup of minced red onion
- One minced garlic clove
- Pinch salt
- One cup of chopped mango
- Two tablespoons of chopped fresh cilantro
- Half tablespoon of freshly squeezed lemon juice

Instructions

1. Combine the onion, mango, cilantro, lemon juice, garlic, and salt in a medium mixing cup.
2. Refrigerate for up to a week in an airtight jar.

13.22 Roasted Root Vegetables

Preparation time-15 minutes| Cook time-35 minutes| Total time-50 minutes| Servings-2|Difficulty-Moderate

Nutritional Facts- Calories: 460; Total Fat: 18g; Total Carbohydrates: 74g; Sugar: 23g; Fiber: 14g; Protein: 6g; Sodium: 760mg

Ingredients

- Half bunch of beets, peeled and cut into 1-inch cubes
- One parsnip, peeled and cut into 1-inch rounds
- One tablespoon of extra-virgin olive oil
- One small sweet potato, peeled and cut into 1-inch cubes
- One and a half carrots, peeled and cut into 1-inch rounds
- Two tablespoons of melted coconut oil
- Half tablespoon of raw honey or maple syrup
- A quarter teaspoon of freshly ground black pepper
- Half teaspoon of salt

Instructions

1. Preheat the oven to 400 degrees Fahrenheit.
2. Line two rimmed baking sheets with parchment paper.
3. Combine the carrots, beets, sweet potatoes, and parsnips in a big mixing bowl. Add the olive oil, coconut oil, salt, honey, and pepper to it. Toss the vegetables in the dressing to cover them.
4. Distribute the vegetables evenly between the two baking sheets, forming a single plate.
5. Bake the vegetables for 10 to 15 minutes on the sheets in a preheated oven. Turn them over until the other side brown. Bake for another 10 to 15 minutes, or until the vegetables are brown and soft. Serve it hot.

13.23 Turmeric Chicken Salad

Preparation time-15 minutes| Cook time-20 minutes| Total time-35 minutes| Servings-2|Difficulty-Easy

Nutritional Facts- Calories: 418; Total Fat: 21g; Total Carbohydrates: 10g; Sugar: 3g; Fiber: 4g; Protein: 46g; Sodium: 759mg

Ingredients

- One tablespoon of extra-virgin olive oil
- One minced garlic clove
- 1/8 teaspoon of ground turmeric
- A quarter cup of plain unsweetened almond yogurt
- Half teaspoon of lemon zest
- Three cups chopped romaine lettuce
- Two boneless skinless chicken breasts
- Half tablespoon of chopped fresh cilantro
- One teaspoon of salt
- A quarter teaspoon of freshly ground black pepper
- Half tablespoon of freshly squeezed lemon juice
- A quarter cup of chopped almonds

Instructions

1. Place the chicken breasts in a shallow baking dish.
2. Whisk together the cilantro, olive oil, garlic, turmeric, salt, and pepper in a small bowl. Using your hands, rub the mixture all over the chicken. Cover the chicken and marinate for at least 30 minutes or overnight in the refrigerator.
3. Preheat the oven to 375 degrees Fahrenheit. Place the baking dish in the preheated oven and bake the chicken for 20 minutes once the oven is warmed. Remove the baking sheet from the oven and put it aside.
4. Whisk together the lemon juice, yogurt, and lemon zest in a big mixing bowl. Toss in the almonds and romaine lettuce to evenly distribute the dressing.

5. Place the salad on a serving platter and serve. Cut the chicken breasts into pieces and place them on top of the lettuce.

13.24 Lentil, Vegetable, and Fruit Bowl

Preparation time-20 minutes| Cook time-0 minutes| Total time-20 minutes| Servings-2|Difficulty-Easy

Nutritional Facts- Calories: 989; Total Fat: 31g; Total Carbohydrates: 151g; Sugar: 16g; Fiber: 35g; Protein: 31g; Sodium: 272mg

Ingredients

- One cup of water
- Half of one (15-ounce) can of lentils, drained and rinsed
- One head radicchio, cored and torn into pieces, divided
- Half cup of red lentils
- One and a half to two cups of cooked brown rice
- Half cup of Chicken Lettuce Wraps sauce
- One small jicama, peeled and cut into thin sticks, divided
- One sliced scallion
- One red Bartlett (or other) ripe pear, cored, quartered, and sliced, divided

Instructions

1. Mix the red lentils and water in a medium mixing bowl. Refrigerate overnight, covered. When you're about to make the salad, drain the lentils.
2. Combine the canned lentils and brown rice in a medium mixing bowl. Half of the Chicken Lettuce Wraps sauce can be added now. Allow for at least 30 minutes of rest time or overnight.
3. In serving bowls, divide the lentil-rice mixture. Add equivalent quantities of soaked and drained red lentils to each dish. Serve with jicama, radicchio, scallions, and pears on the side.
4. Drizzle some of the leftover Chicken Lettuce Wraps sauce over each one.

13.25 Roasted Cauliflower with Almond Sauce

Preparation time-15 minutes| Cook time-20 minutes| Total time-35 minutes| Servings-2|Difficulty-Easy

Nutritional Facts- Calories: 277; Total Fat: 23g; Total Carbohydrates: 15g; Sugar: 6g; Fiber: 4g; Protein: 7g; Sodium: 945mg

Ingredients

- Two tablespoons of extra-virgin olive oil
- One teaspoon of salt, divided
- Half cup of plain unsweetened almond yogurt
- Half sliced scallion
- Half tablespoon of chopped fresh parsley

- Half tablespoon of maple syrup
- Half head cauliflower, cut into florets
- A quarter teaspoon of a teaspoon of ground turmeric
- A quarter teaspoon of freshly ground black pepper, divided
- Two tablespoons of almond butter
- One minced garlic clove
- Half tablespoon of freshly squeezed lemon juice

Instructions

1. Preheat the oven to 400 degrees Fahrenheit.
2. Combine the cauliflower, turmeric, olive oil, pepper, and salt in a wide mixing bowl.
3. Arrange the seasoned cauliflower in a single layer on a rimmed baking sheet. Roast for 20 to 30 minutes, or until the cauliflower is gently browned and moist, on a baking sheet in a preheated oven.
4. Combine the yogurt, almond butter, garlic, scallions, parsley, maple syrup, lemon juice, and salt and pepper in a processor. Purée until entirely smooth.
5. Spread the almond sauce over the roasted cauliflower in a serving bowl.

13.26 Cauliflower Purée

Preparation time-15 minutes| Cook time-10 minutes| Total time-25 minutes| Servings-2|Difficulty-Easy

Nutritional Facts- Calories: 117; Total Fat: 11g; Total Carbohydrates: 6g; Sugar: 3g; Fiber: 2g; Protein: 2g; Sodium: 1187mg

Ingredients

- One garlic clove
- 1/8 teaspoon of freshly ground black pepper
- Half tablespoon of extra-virgin olive oil
- Half head cauliflower, broken into florets
- One teaspoon of salt, divided
- A quarter cup of coconut milk

Instructions

1. Using high heat, bring a big pot of water to a boil. Add the garlic clove, cauliflower, and salt to it. Cook for 5 minutes, or until the cauliflower is soft.
2. Drain the cauliflower and place it in a large mixing bowl with the garlic clove. Using a potato masher, mash the cauliflower until they are smooth.
3. Toss the mashed cauliflower with salt, pepper, and coconut milk. Mix everything together thoroughly.
4. Drizzle a little olive oil over the purée in a serving bowl.

13.27 Green Beans with Crispy Shallots

Preparation time-10 minutes| Cook time-15 minutes| Total time-25 minutes| Servings-2|Difficulty-Easy

Nutritional Facts- Calories: 146; Total Fat: 13g; Total Carbohydrates: 9g; Sugar: 2g; Fiber: 4g; Protein: 2g; Sodium: 475mg

Ingredients

- Half pound of trimmed green beans
- Half thinly sliced large shallot
- Freshly ground black pepper
- Half teaspoon of sea salt, plus additional for seasoning
- Two tablespoons of extra-virgin olive oil
- Half tablespoon of chopped fresh tarragon

Instructions

1. Over high heat, bring a big pot of water to a boil.
2. Add a teaspoon of sea salt into the boiling water before adding the beans. Cook for 5 minutes, or before they develop a vibrant green color.
3. Drain and pass the beans to a serving bowl.
4. Heat the olive oil in a small saucepan over medium heat. Add the shallots once the oil is hot. Cook for 1 to 2 minutes, or until the browning begins.
5. Serve the green beans with the shallots on top. Season with pepper and sea salt after adding the tarragon.

13.28 Roasted Sweet Potatoes and Pineapple

Preparation time-15 minutes| Cook time-25 minutes| Total time-40 minutes| Servings-2|Difficulty-Moderate

Nutritional Facts- Calories: 230; Total Fat: 11g; Total Carbohydrates: 34g; Sugar: 5g; Fiber: 5g; Protein: 2g; Sodium: 591mg

Ingredients

- One large sweet potato, or yams, peeled and cut into 1/2-inch pieces
- One teaspoon of curry powder
- Two tablespoons of freshly ground black pepper
- One and a half tablespoons of coconut oil
- Half cup of fresh pineapple, cut into 1/2-inch pieces
- One teaspoon of salt

Instructions

1. Preheat the oven to 400 degrees Fahrenheit.
2. Microwave the coconut oil for around a minute on high in a microwave-safe bowl.

3. Combine the pineapple and sweet potatoes in a big mixing bowl. Add the molten coconut oil, salt, curry powder, and pepper. Toss all around.
4. Fill a rimmed baking sheet halfway with the mixture. Roast for 20 to 25 minutes, or until the sweet potatoes are soft, on a baking sheet in a preheated oven.
5. Serve immediately, hot.

Chapter 14-Dessert Recipes

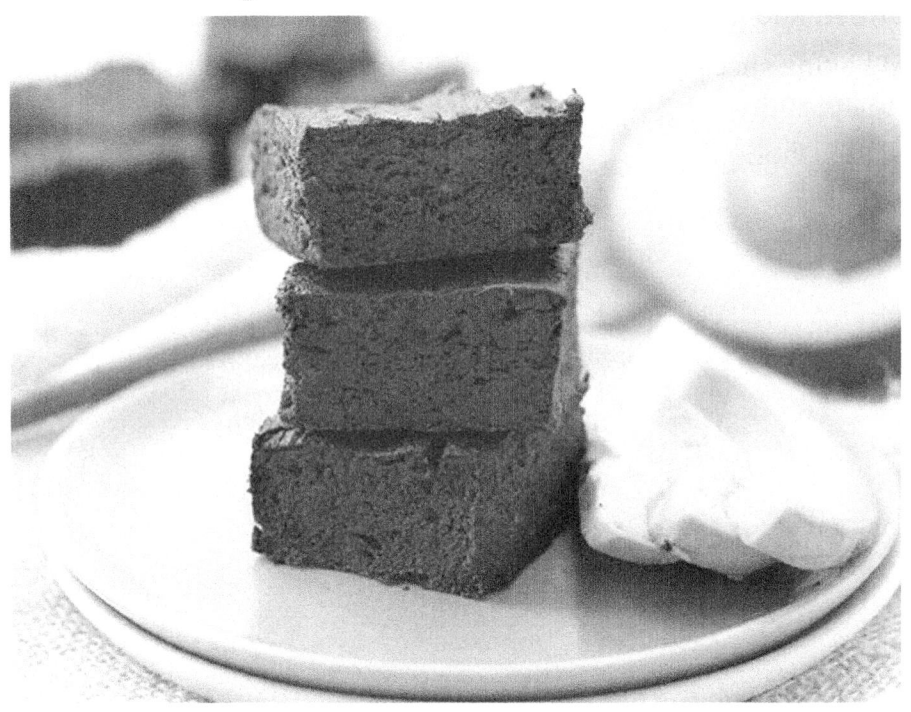

14.1 Sweet Spiced Pecans

Preparation time-5 minutes| Cook time-17 minutes| Total time-22 minutes| Servings-2|Difficulty-Easy

Nutritional Facts- Calories: 323; Total Fat: 30g; Total Carbs: 14g; Sugar: 10g; Fiber: 4g; Protein: 3g; Sodium: 181mg

Ingredients

- Two tablespoons of packed brown sugar
- Half teaspoon of ground cinnamon
- A pinch of sea salt
- Half cup of pecan halves
- One and a half tablespoons of unsalted butter, melted
- A quarter teaspoon of ground nutmeg

Instructions

1. Preheat the oven to 350 degrees Fahrenheit.
2. Using parchment paper, line a rimmed baking dish.
3. Toss the brown sugar, pecans, butter, nutmeg, cinnamon, and salt together in a medium mixing dish. On the prepared mat, spread the nuts in a single layer.
4. Bake for 15–17 minutes, or until the nuts are fragrant.

14.2 Honeyed Apple Cinnamon Compote

Preparation time-15 minutes| Cook time-10 minutes| Total time-25 minutes| Servings-2|Difficulty-Easy

Nutritional Facts- Calories: 247; Total Fat: <1g; Total Carbs: 66g; Sugar: 54g; Fiber: 9g; Protein: 1g; Sodium: 63mg

Ingredients

- Two tablespoons of apple juice
- Three peeled, cored, and chopped apples
- Two tablespoons of honey
- Pinch sea salt
- Half teaspoon of ground cinnamon

Instructions

1. Combine all of the ingredients in a big pot over medium-high heat.
2. Cook, stirring regularly, for around 10 minutes, or until the apples are already chunky yet saucy.

14.3 Cranberry Compote

Preparation time-5 minutes| Cook time-15 minutes| Total time-20 minutes| Servings-2|Difficulty-Easy

Nutritional Facts- Calories: 172; Total Fat: <1g; Total Carbs: 39g; Sugar: 30g; Fiber: 6g; Protein: 1g; Sodium: 1mg

Ingredients

- Two tablespoons of honey
- Two cups of fresh cranberries
- Half tablespoon of grated fresh ginger
- Zest of half orange
- Juice of one orange

Instructions

1. Combine the cranberries, orange juice, ginger, honey, and orange zest in a big pot over medium-high heat. Get the water to a simmer.
2. Cook, stirring regularly, for around 10 minutes, or until the cranberries pop and shape a sauce.
3. Refrigerate or eat right away.

14.4 Coconut Rice with Blueberries

Preparation time-15 minutes| Cook time-10 minutes| Total time-25 minutes| Servings-2|Difficulty-Easy

Nutritional Facts- Calories: 469; Total Fat: 25g; Total Carbs: 60g; Sugar: 19g; Fiber: 5g; Protein: 6g; Sodium: 76mg

Ingredients

- Half cup of fresh blueberries
- Half teaspoon of ground ginger
- One cup of cooked brown rice
- Half of one (14-ounce) can of full-fat coconut milk
- Two tablespoons of sugar
- Pinch sea salt

Instructions

1. Combine the blueberries, coconut milk, ginger, sugar, and salt in a big pot over medium-high heat. Cook, stirring continuously, for around 7 minutes, or until the blueberries soften.
2. Include the rice and mix well. Cook, sometimes stirring, for around 3 minutes, or until the rice is thoroughly cooked.

14.5 Greek Yogurt with Blueberries, Nuts, and Honey

Preparation time-5 minutes| Cook time-0 minutes| Total time-5 minutes| Servings-2|Difficulty-Easy

Nutritional Facts- Calories: 457; Total Fat: 18g; Total Carbs: 62g; Sugar: 54g; Fiber: 3g; Protein: 15g; Sodium: 213mg

Ingredients

- One cup of blueberries
- A quarter cup of honey
- One and a half cups of unsweetened plain Greek yogurt
- A quarter cup of chopped mixed nuts

Instructions

1. Divide the yogurt into two cups.
2. Drizzle with honey after adding the blueberries and nuts.

14.6 Maple-Glazed Pears with Hazelnuts

Preparation time-10 minutes| Cook time-20 minutes| Total time-15 minutes| Servings-2|Difficulty-Easy

Nutritional Facts- Calories: 286; Total Fat: 3g; Total Carbs: 67g; Sugar: 50g; Fiber: 7g; Protein: 2g; Sodium: 9mg

Ingredients

- Half cup of apple juice
- Two pears, peeled, cored, and quartered lengthwise
- A quarter cup of pure maple syrup
- Two tablespoons of chopped hazelnuts

- Half tablespoon of grated fresh ginger

Instructions

1. Combine the apple juice and pears in a big pot over medium-high flame. Reduce the heat to medium-low and bring to a simmer. Cook, covered, for 15 to 20 minutes, or until the pears are tender.
2. When the pears are poaching, mix the maple syrup and ginger in a small saucepan over medium-high heat. Bring to a low boil, stirring sometimes. Allow the syrup to cool in the pan after removing it from the sun.
3. Break the pears from the poaching solvent with a slotted spoon and sprinkle with maple syrup. Serve with hazelnuts on top.

14.7 Green Tea–Poached Pears

Preparation time-5 minutes| Cook time-15 minutes| Total time-20 minutes| Servings-2|Difficulty-Easy

Nutritional Facts- Calories: 190; Total Fat: <1g; Total Carbs: 50g; Sugar: 38g; Fiber: 7g; Protein: <1g; Sodium: 4mg

Ingredients

- One cup of strongly brewed green tea
- Half tablespoon of grated fresh ginger
- Two pears, peeled, cored, and quartered lengthwise
- Two tablespoons of honey

Instructions

1. Combine the tea, honey, pears, and ginger in a big pot over medium-high flame. Bring to a low boil, then reduce to low heat.
2. Reduce the heat to medium-low, cover, and let the pears soften for around 15 minutes.
3. Serve the pears with a spoonful of the poaching liquid on top.

14.8 Blueberry Ambrosia

Preparation time-15 minutes| Cook time-0 minutes| Total time-15 minutes| Servings-2|Difficulty-Easy

Nutritional Facts- Calories: 387; Total Fat: 21g; Total Carbs: 46g; Sugar: 31g; Fiber: 11g; Protein: 4g; Sodium: 17mg

Ingredients

- One tablespoon of honey
- Half of one (14-ounce) can of full-fat coconut milk, chilled
- One pint of fresh blueberries
- Half peeled, cored, and chopped apple
- One pint of fresh raspberries

Instructions

1. Open the cooled coconut milk can and scrape the solids from the surface into a big mixing cup. Any remaining water could be discarded.
2. Combine the coconut milk and honey in a mixing bowl.
3. To coat the raspberries, blueberries, and apple with the coconut milk, gently stir them in.

14.9 Easy Peanut Butter Balls

Preparation time-15 minutes| Cook time-0 minutes| Total time-15 minutes| Servings-6 balls |Difficulty-Easy

Nutritional Facts- Calories: 147; Total Fat: 8g; Total Carbs: 17g; Sugar: 15g; Fiber: 1g; Protein: 4g; Sodium: 71mg

Ingredients

- One tablespoon of unsalted butter softened
- A quarter cup of creamy peanut butter
- A quarter cup of powdered sugar
- A quarter teaspoon of vanilla extract
- Two and a half tablespoons of unsweetened cocoa powder

Instructions

1. Stir together the butter, peanut butter, cocoa powder, powdered sugar, and vanilla in a medium mixing bowl until well mixed.
2. Place the mixture on a parchment paper-lined tray and roll it into six balls. Refrigerate or eat right away.

14.10 Chocolate–Almond Butter Mousse

Preparation time-15 minutes| Cook time-0 minutes| Total time-15 minutes| Servings-2|Difficulty-Easy

Nutritional Facts- Calories: 271; Total Fat: 21g; Total Carbs: 23g; Sugar: 12g; Fiber: 7g; Protein: 2g; Sodium: 70mg

Ingredients

- Two tablespoons of almond butter
- Two tablespoons of unsweetened cocoa powder
- Pinch sea salt
- One peeled and pitted avocado
- Two tablespoons of lite coconut milk
- Two tablespoons of pure maple syrup

Instructions

1. In a blender or food processor, combine all the ingredients together.
2. Process until smooth.

3. Pour in the glasses and let them cool in the refrigerator before eating them.

14.11 Melon with Berry- Yogurt Sauce

Preparation time-15 minutes| Cook time-0 minutes| Total time-15 minutes| Servings-2|Difficulty-Easy

Nutritional Facts- Calories: 76; Total Fat: 4g; Total Carbohydrates: 11g; Sugar: 5g; Fiber: 6g; Protein: 1g; Sodium: 37mg

Ingredients

- One pint of fresh raspberries
- Half cantaloupe, peeled and sliced
- A quarter teaspoon of vanilla extract
- A quarter cup of toasted coconut
- Half cup of plain coconut or almond yogurt

Instructions

1. On a serving tray, arrange the melon slices.
2. Mash the berries with the vanilla in a bit of dish. Stir in the yogurt until it is thoroughly combined.
3. Sprinkle the coconut over the melon slices and top with the berry-yogurt mixture.

14.12 Roasted Peaches with Raspberry Sauce and Coconut Cream

Preparation time-15 minutes| Cook time-15 minutes| Total time-30 minutes| Servings-2|Difficulty-Easy

Nutritional Facts- Calories: 261; Total Fat: 16g; Total Carbohydrates: 31g; Sugar: 25g; Fiber: 6g; Protein: 3g; Sodium: 5mg

Ingredients

- One tablespoon of melted coconut oil
- Two halved ripe peaches
- Half of one (10-ounce) bag frozen no-added-sugar raspberries, thawed
- One tablespoon of chopped pistachios
- A quarter cup of Coconut Cream

Instructions

1. Preheat the oven to 400 degrees Fahrenheit.
2. Place the peaches in a shallow baking dish and brush them with the melted coconut oil.
3. Roast the peaches for 10 to 15 minutes or until they start to brown.
4. Purée the raspberries in a food processor as the peaches are roasting. If you don't want your raspberry sauce to have seeds, filter it via a fine-mesh strainer.
5. Place the peaches cut-side up on a serving platter to eat. Serve with a dollop of Coconut Cream, a drizzle of raspberry sauce, and a sprinkling of pistachios on top.

14.13 Cherry Ice Cream

Preparation time-10 minutes| Cook time-0 minutes| Total time-10 minutes| Servings-2|Difficulty-Easy

Nutritional Facts- Calories: 82; Total Fat: 2g; Total Carbohydrates: 14g; Sugar: 12g; Fiber: 2g; Protein: 1g; Sodium: 121mg

Ingredients

- One and a half cups of unsweetened almond milk
- A quarter teaspoon of almond extract
- Half of one (10-ounce) package of frozen no-added-sugar cherries
- Half teaspoon of vanilla extract

Instructions

1. Combine the almond milk, vanilla extract, cherries, and almond extract in a blender or food processor. Process until almost smooth, with a few cherry chunks appropriate.
2. Fill a pot with the mixture and close it tightly. Until serving, make sure it is fully frozen.

14.14 Blueberry Crisp

Preparation time-15 minutes| Cook time-20 minutes| Total time-35 minutes| Servings-2|Difficulty-Easy

Nutritional Facts- Calories: 497; Total Fat: 33g; Total Carbohydrates: 51g; Sugar: 26g; Fiber: 7g; Protein: 5g; Sodium: 42mg

Ingredients

- Half quart of fresh blueberries
- Juice of half lemon
- Half cup of gluten-free rolled oats
- A quarter cup of coconut oil, melted, plus additional for brushing
- Two tablespoons of maple syrup
- One teaspoon of lemon zest
- A quarter teaspoon of ground cinnamon
- Pinch salt
- A quarter cup of chopped pecans

Instructions

1. Preheat the oven to 350 degrees Fahrenheit.
2. Melt the coconut oil in a small baking dish. In a mixing bowl, combine the blueberries, lemon juice, maple syrup, and lemon zest.
3. Combine the oats, cinnamon, pecans, half cup melted coconut oil, and salt in a shallow mixing dish. To uniformly spread the coconut oil, thoroughly combine the ingredients. Over the fruit, sprinkle the oat mixture.

4. Bake the dish for 20 minutes, or until the oats, are finely browned.

14.15 Grilled Pineapple with Chocolate Ganache

Preparation time-30 minutes| Cook time-15 minutes| Total time-45 minutes| Servings-2|Difficulty-Moderate

Nutritional Facts- Calories: 462; Total Fat: 23g; Total Carbohydrates: 61g; Sugar: 48g; Fiber: 2g; Protein: 5g; Sodium: 5mg

Ingredients

For the ganache

- One cup of semi-sweet or bittersweet chocolate morsels
- A quarter cup of coconut milk

For the pineapple

- Half tablespoon of coconut oil, melted
- Half teaspoon of chopped fresh rosemary
- Half pineapple, peeled, cored, and cut into eight wedges
- Half tablespoon of coconut sugar

Instructions

To make the ganache

1. Add the coconut milk to a medium saucepan over medium-high flame. Heat the milk until it scalds only a bit (tiny bubbles or foam will begin to collect around the perimeter of the pan).
2. Take the pan off the heat and stir in the chocolate. Allow for 1 minute of resting time.
3. Whisk the paste until it's silky smooth.

To make the pineapple

1. Preheat an indoor stove-top barbecue to a high temperature.
2. Melt the coconut oil and brush it on the pineapple wedges.
3. Grill for 1 to 2 minutes per hand, or before grill marks show on both sides.
4. Sprinkle the coconut sugar and rosemary over the pineapple on a serving platter.
5. Serve with ganache on top.

14.16 Chocolate-Avocado Mousse with Sea Salt

Preparation time-10 minutes| Cook time-5 minutes| Total time-15 minutes refrigeration time excluded| Servings-2|Difficulty-Easy

Nutritional Facts- Calories: 653; Total Fat: 47g; Total Carbohydrates: 56g; Sugar: 42g; Fiber: 9g; Protein: 7g; Sodium: 113mg

Ingredients

- Two tablespoons of coconut milk
- One ripe avocado

- Pinch sea salt
- Four ounces of chopped bittersweet chocolate
- One tablespoon of coconut oil
- Two tablespoons of raw honey or maple syrup

Instructions

1. Combine the coconut milk, chocolate, and coconut oil in a tiny heavy saucepan over low heat. Cook, stirring continuously for 2 to 3 minutes, or until the chocolate melts.
2. Combine the honey and avocado in a food processor. Process the molten chocolate until it is almost smooth.
3. Serve the mousse in serving bowls with a layer of sea salt on top.
4. Until serving, chill for at least 30 minutes.

14.17 Fruit and Walnut Crumble

Preparation time-15 minutes| Cook time-20 minutes| Total time-35 minutes| Servings-2|Difficulty-Easy

Nutritional Facts- Calories: 335; Total Fat: 19g; Total Carbohydrates: 42g; Sugar: 32g; Fiber: 6g; Protein: 6g; Sodium: 32mg

Ingredients

For the topping

- Two tablespoons of coarsely chopped hazelnuts
- Half cup of coarsely chopped walnuts
- Half tablespoon of ghee or melted coconut oil
- Pinch salt
- Half teaspoon of ground cinnamon

For the filling

- One halved fresh fig
- A quarter cup of coconut sugar, raw honey, or maple syrup
- Half teaspoon of vanilla extract
- Half cup of fresh blueberries
- One pitted and sliced nectarine
- One teaspoon of lemon zest

Instructions

To make the topping

1. Combine the hazelnuts, walnuts, cinnamon, ghee, and salt in a shallow mixing cup, then set it aside.

To make the filling

1. Preheat the oven to 375 degrees Fahrenheit.
2. Combine the figs, blueberries, nectarines, lemon zest, coconut sugar, and vanilla in a medium mixing bowl.
3. Divide the fruit into two single-serving oven-safe bowls or ramekins.
4. Distribute the nut topping evenly among the servings.
5. Bake the bowls for 15 to 20 minutes, or until the nuts are golden brown and the fruit is bubbling.

14.18 Coconut Ice Cream Sandwiches

Preparation time-45 minutes| Cook time-15 minutes| Total time-1 hour refrigeration time excluded| Servings-2|Difficulty-Hard

Nutritional Facts- Calories: 673; Total Fat: 53g; Total Carbohydrates: 48g; Sugar: 42g; Fiber: 2g; Protein: 5g; Sodium: 538mg

Ingredients

For the coconut ice cream

- Two tablespoons of coconut sugar
- One teaspoon of vanilla extract
- Two cups of full-fat coconut milk

For the cookies

- One tablespoon of coconut sugar
- A pinch of baking soda
- Two tablespoons coconut oil, melted and cooled slightly
- One cup of almond flour
- Half teaspoon of salt
- Two tablespoons of ground cardamom
- Two tablespoons of maple syrup
- Half teaspoon of vanilla extract
- Half tablespoon of almond milk

For the finished ice cream sandwiches

- A quarter cup of shredded coconut

Instructions

To make the coconut ice cream

1. Combine the coconut sugar and coconut milk in a big saucepan over medium heat. Cook, stirring vigorously for about 5 minutes, or until the sugar melts. Take the pan off the heat and add the vanilla extract.

2. Refrigerate the mixture for at least 4 hours, or up to 24 hours.
3. Make the ice cream as per the ice cream maker's manufacturer's directions.
4. Put the ice cream in an airtight jar and freeze it.

To make the cookies

1. Preheat the oven to 325 degrees Fahrenheit.
2. Line two baking sheets with parchment paper.
3. Combine the coconut sugar, almond flour, baking soda, salt, and cardamom in a medium mixing cup.
4. Combine the almond milk, maple syrup, coconut oil, and vanilla extract in a mixing bowl. In a large mixing bowl, combine all of the ingredients until a dense dough emerges.
5. Place scoops of dough on prepared sheets with a spoon, leaving about 2 inches for each cookie. Four to six cookies should be able to be made from the dough. Using the palm or the back of a spoon, gently flatten the cookies.
6. Bake the sheets for 10 to 12 minutes, or until golden brown, in a preheated oven. Before preparing the ice cream sandwiches, let the cookies cool down.

To assemble the ice cream sandwiches

1. Place a generous scoop of coconut ice cream on one cookie's bottom and cover it with another cookie, softly pushing it together. Cover the cookies in plastic wrap and ice before ready to snack.
2. When ready to eat, press shredded coconut around the sides of each sandwich in the ice cream.

14.19 Chocolate-Cherry Clusters

Preparation time-15 minutes| Cook time-0 minutes| Total time-15 minutes| Servings-4 clusters |Difficulty-Easy

Nutritional Facts- Calories: 198; Total Fat: 13g; Total Carbohydrates: 18g; Sugar: 12g; Fiber: 4g; Protein: 4g; Sodium: 58mg

Ingredients

- Half tablespoon of coconut oil
- Two tablespoons of dried cherries
- A quarter cup of dark chocolate (60 percent cocoa or higher), chopped
- Half cup of roasted salted almonds

Instructions

1. Wax paper can be used to line a rimmed baking sheet.
2. Stir the coconut oil and chocolate together in a double boiler until smooth and molten.
3. Remove the pan from the heat and add the cherries and almonds.
4. Drop clusters onto wax paper by the spoon. Refrigerate until fully set.
5. Refrigerate until transferring to an airtight bag.

14.20 Gluten-Free Oat and Fruit Bars

Preparation time-15 minutes| Cook time-45 minutes| Total time-1 hour| Servings-4 bars| Difficulty-Hard

Nutritional Facts- Calories: 144; Total Fat: 7g; Total Carbohydrates: 19g; Sugar: 8g; Fiber: 2g; Protein: 3g; Sodium: 3mg

Ingredients

- Two tablespoons of maple syrup
- One mashed medium ripe banana
- Half cup of old-fashioned rolled oats
- One and a half tablespoons of oat flour
- Half teaspoon of vanilla extract
- 1/8 teaspoon of ground cloves
- Cooking spray
- Two tablespoons of almond or sunflower butter
- One and a half tablespoons of dried cranberries
- Two tablespoons of shredded coconut
- One and a half tablespoon of ground flaxseed
- 1/8 teaspoon of ground cinnamon

Instructions

1. Preheat the oven to 400 degrees Fahrenheit.
2. Cover an 8-by-8-inch square pan with cooking spray after lining it with parchment paper or aluminum foil.
3. Combine the almond butter, maple syrup, and bananas in a medium mixing dish. Mix, so it is well combined.
4. Combine the cranberries, coconut, oats, oat flour, cinnamon, vanilla, flaxseed, and cloves in a large mixing bowl. Mix well.
5. The mixture would be moist and sticky when spooned into the prepared pan. Spread the mixture uniformly using an oiled spatula.
6. Bake for 40 to 45 minutes, or until the surface is dry and a toothpick inserted in the center comes out clean in a preheated oven. Until cutting through bars, allow cooling fully.

14.21 Pumpkin Coconut Pie with Almond Crust

Preparation time-15 minutes| Cook time-55 minutes| Total time-1 hour 10 minutes plus refrigeration time | Servings-2|Difficulty-Hard

Nutritional Facts- Calories: 144; Total Fat: 7g; Total Carbohydrates: 19g; Sugar: 8g; Fiber: 2g; Protein: 3g; Sodium: 3mg

Ingredients

For the crust

- One and a half tablespoons of arrowroot powder
- A quarter teaspoon of sea salt
- A quarter cup of almond meal
- A quarter teaspoon of baking powder
- 1/8 teaspoon of xanthan gum
- One and a half tablespoons of cold water plus more as per requirement
- One tablespoon of coconut oil

For the filling

- One tablespoon of ground flaxseed
- A quarter cup of coconut milk
- A quarter teaspoon of ground cinnamon
- 1/8 teaspoon of sea salt
- A pinch of ground cloves or allspice
- One tablespoon of hot water plus more as per requirement
- Half cup of pumpkin puree
- Two tablespoons of agave nectar or maple syrup
- A quarter teaspoon of ground ginger
- 1/8 teaspoon of freshly grated or ground nutmeg

Instructions

1. To create the crust, combine the arrowroot powder, almond meal, salt, baking powder, and xanthan gum in a big mixing bowl and stir well. With a fork or pastry knife, blend in the coconut oil until the mixture is crumbly. Stir in the water in a slow, steady stream before the dough forms a ball. Refrigerate for around 1 hour after dividing into two equal balls and wrap in plastic wrap.
2. Preheat oven to 375 degrees Fahrenheit.
3. To form the filling, combine the hot water and flaxseed in a small bowl. Allow 10 minutes for the mixture to rest before transferring to a wide mixing bowl. In a large mixing bowl, combine the coconut milk, nutmeg, pumpkin puree, agave, ginger, cinnamon, salt, and cloves.
4. Roll out one dough ball between two sheets of waxed paper to a width of around 10 inches. Move the dough to a 9-inch pie pan and gently push it into shape. Heat the crust in the oven for 8 to 10 minutes.
5. It's possible that the crust would start to brown somewhat. Bake for 35 to 45 minutes, or until the filling no longer jiggles, after pouring the filling into the crust. If the crust begins to brown so much, you can need to wrap foil around the sides.
6. Allow the pie to cool fully before eating, then refrigerate for 2 to 3 hours.

14.22 Mixed Berry Walnut Crumble

Preparation time-10 minutes| Cook time-55 minutes| Total time-1 hour 5 minutes| Servings-2|Difficulty-Hard

Nutritional Facts- Calories: 198; Total Fat: 13g; Total Carbohydrates: 18g; Sugar: 12g; Fiber: 4g; Protein: 4g; Sodium: 58mg

Ingredients

For the filling

- Two tablespoons of agave nectar
- A quarter teaspoon of ground cinnamon
- Two and a half cups of fresh or frozen mixed berries
- Half tablespoons of arrowroot powder
- A quarter teaspoon of ground nutmeg

For the crumble

- A quarter cup of chopped walnuts
- One and a half tablespoon of agave nectar
- Half cup of certified gluten-free oats
- Two tablespoons of brown rice flour
- A quarter teaspoon of ground cinnamon
- A quarter cup of coconut oil, plus more for oiling dish
- A quarter teaspoon of ground allspice

Instructions

1. Preheat oven to 350 degrees Fahrenheit. Using coconut oil, lightly oil a 9-by-13-inch baking dish.
2. To create the filling, add the agave, berries, cinnamon, arrowroot powder, and nutmeg in a big mixing bowl and toss until evenly covered. Bake for 35 minutes after transferring to the baking dish and covering with foil.
3. In a medium mixing dish, combine the oats, cinnamon, flour, walnuts, agave, and allspice to create the topping. With a fork or pastry knife, blend in the coconut oil until the mixture is crumbly.
4. Cover the fruit filling with the filling. Bake for 20 minutes, uncovered, or until the topping is golden brown. Until eating, enable the crumble to cool slightly.

14.23 Rustic Pear and Fig Crostatas

Preparation time-10 minutes| Cook time-30 minutes| Total time-40 minutes| Servings-2|Difficulty-Moderate

Nutritional Facts- Calories: 201; Total Fat: 12g; Total Carbohydrates: 20g; Sugar: 13g; Fiber: 8g; Protein: 4g; Sodium: 66mg

Ingredients

- Half of one large thinly sliced unpeeled pear
- A quarter teaspoon of sea salt
- One tablespoon of agave nectar or maple syrup
- Two tablespoons of honey
- Three to four fresh figs, cut into 1⁄2-inch chunks
- One cup of brown rice flour, plus more for dusting
- A quarter cup plus three tablespoons of coconut oil
- One to Two tablespoons of cold water

Instructions

1. Preheat oven to 350 degrees Fahrenheit.
2. In a medium dish, combine the figs and pear and set aside.
3. Combine the salt and flour in a small bowl. Beat the coconut oil in the bowl of a stand mixer equipped with the paddle attachment for 1 minute or until saturated. Slowly apply the flour mixture to the mixer at low speed before it is completely incorporated. Continue to beat in the agave and cold water before a smooth dough forms.
4. Make six fair balls out of the dough. One ball should be flattened and floured. Make a 4-inch disc out of the dough. 2 big spoonsful of the fruit mixture should be placed in the middle, with a 1/2-inch border of dough around the sides. Pull the dough up along the fruit's sides, leaving the middle unprotected. Using the remaining dough balls and berries, repeat the process.
5. Move the crostatas and parchment to a baking pan with care. Drizzle honey over the tops of each crostata and bake for 25 minutes, or until the pears are soft and the crusts are golden brown.

14.24 So-Easy Coconut Mango Sorbet

Preparation time-15 minutes| Cook time-0 minutes| Total time-15 minutes plus refrigeration time | Servings-2|Difficulty-Easy

Nutritional Facts- Calories: 210; Total Fat: 12g; Total Carbohydrates: 18g; Sugar: 14g; Fiber: 5g; Protein: 6g; Sodium: 61mg

Ingredients

- Half cup of coconut milk
- A quarter teaspoon of vanilla extract
- Half of one (10-ounce) bag of frozen mangoes
- A quarter cup of hazelnut or almond milk

Instructions

1. Blend all the ingredients until smooth in a food processor or blender.
2. Serve right away or place in the freezer until the sorbet reaches the perfect consistency.

14.25 Baked Pears or Apples with Cashew Cream

Preparation time-15 minutes| Cook time-1 hour| Total time- 1 hour and 15 minutes| Servings- 2|Difficulty- Hard

Nutritional Facts- Calories: 208; Total Fat: 16g; Total Carbohydrates: 15g; Sugar: 15g; Fiber: 7g; Protein: 3g; Sodium: 55mg

Ingredients

- Half cup of water
- One large unpeeled pear or apple, cored and halved
- One to Two tablespoons of ground cinnamon
- Half cup of raw cashews
- One tablespoon of agave nectar

Instructions

1. Preheat oven to 375 degrees Fahrenheit.
2. In a medium baking dish, place the pears or apples face down. Half a cup of water should be added to the bowl, which should be covered with foil and baked for 45 minutes. Uncover the apple, sprinkle it with cinnamon, drizzle it with agave, and bake for another 5 minutes, or until tender but not mushy.
3. In the meanwhile, pulse the cashews in a food processor until smooth. Slowly drizzle in a quarter cup of water until the cream is the consistency you like.
4. Fill bowls halfway with berries and a heaping spoonful of cashew milk. Heat the dish before serving.

14.26 Strawberry Rhubarb Crumble

Preparation time-10 minutes| Cook time-1 hour| Total time-1 hour 10 minutes| Servings- 2|Difficulty-Hard

Nutritional Facts- Calories: 199; Total Fat: 17g; Total Carbohydrates: 19g; Sugar: 18g; Fiber: 9g; Protein: 3g; Sodium: 86mg

Ingredients

For the filling

- Half tablespoon of arrowroot powder
- One tablespoon of coconut palm sugar
- A pinch of sea salt
- One cup of strawberries, hulled and quartered
- A quarter-pound of trimmed rhubarb, cut into 1/4-inch-thick pieces

For the crumble

- Two tablespoons of coconut flour
- A quarter teaspoon of baking powder

- A pinch of sea salt
- One tablespoon of hot water
- Two tablespoons of coconut palm sugar
- One tablespoon of white rice flour
- Two tablespoons of ground cinnamon
- Two tablespoons of certified gluten-free rolled oats
- A quarter tablespoon of ground flaxseed
- One tablespoon of melted coconut oil
- Half tablespoon of agave nectar or maple syrup

Instructions

1. Preheat oven to 375 degrees Fahrenheit.
2. To create the filling, whisk together the arrowroot powder, coconut palm sugar, and salt in a medium mixing cup. Toss in the strawberries and rhubarb when evenly covered. In a 10-inch pie plate, spread the fruit and put it aside.
3. To create the topping, whisk together the flours, coconut palm sugar, cinnamon, baking powder, and salt in a medium mixing bowl.
4. Add the oats and mix well.
5. Combine the hot water and flaxseed in a shallow bowl. Allow 10 minutes for the mixture to rest before adding it to the dry ingredients. Add the agave nectar. Knead the ingredients together with your hands until well mixed. Using a fork, uniformly distribute the topping over the berries. Drizzle the coconut oil over the topping in an even layer.
6. Bake the crumble for 45 to 50 minutes, or until the fruit is bubbling and the topping has become golden brown. Allow cooling for a few minutes before serving.

14.27 Vanilla Wafer Pudding

Preparation time-15 minutes| Cook time-0 minutes| Total time-15 minutes| Servings-2|Difficulty-Easy

Nutritional Facts- Calories: 218; Total Fat: 17g; Total Carbohydrates: 20g; Sugar: 19g; Fiber: 3g; Protein: 8g; Sodium: 66mg

Ingredients

- Half ripe banana
- A quarter cup of coconut milk
- One tablespoon of agave nectar
- One cup of raw macadamia nuts
- 3/4 cup of water
- Two teaspoons of chia seeds

Instructions

1. In a food processor, combine all of the ingredients and process until smooth.
2. Refrigerate for at least 2 hours or overnight in an airtight container.

14.28 No-Bake Peach Pie

Preparation time-25 minutes| Cook time-0 minutes| Total time-25 minutes| Servings-2|Difficulty-Easy

Nutritional Facts- Calories: 201; Total Fat: 18g; Total Carbohydrates: 15g; Sugar: 14g; Fiber: 5g; Protein: 7g; Sodium: 68mg

Ingredients

For the crust

- ¾ cup of pitted dates
- A quarter teaspoon of sea salt
- Three cups of raw walnuts
- One tablespoon of ground cinnamon

For the filling

- Half cup of creamed coconut, chopped into chunks
- Two tablespoons of maple syrup
- Three peeled and thinly sliced ripe peaches
- ¾ cup of hot water
- Two cups of raw cashews
- Seeds from one vanilla bean

Instructions

1. To create the crust, in a food processor, mix the cinnamon, dates, walnuts, and salt and pulse until finely chopped and well mixed.
2. Scrape the batter into a 9-inch pie pan that has been lightly oiled with coconut oil. Press the crust onto the pan's rim, raising it back to the top edge all over. Before you begin, make sure the food processor is clean.
3. To create the filling, combine the hot water and creamed coconut in a food processor and process until smooth, around 5 minutes. Blend until smooth with the maple syrup, cashews, and vanilla bean seeds.
4. Evenly spread the cream onto the crust. Over the cream filling, arrange the peaches in a circular shape. Serve it right away.

Chapter 15-Dressings and Sauces Recipes

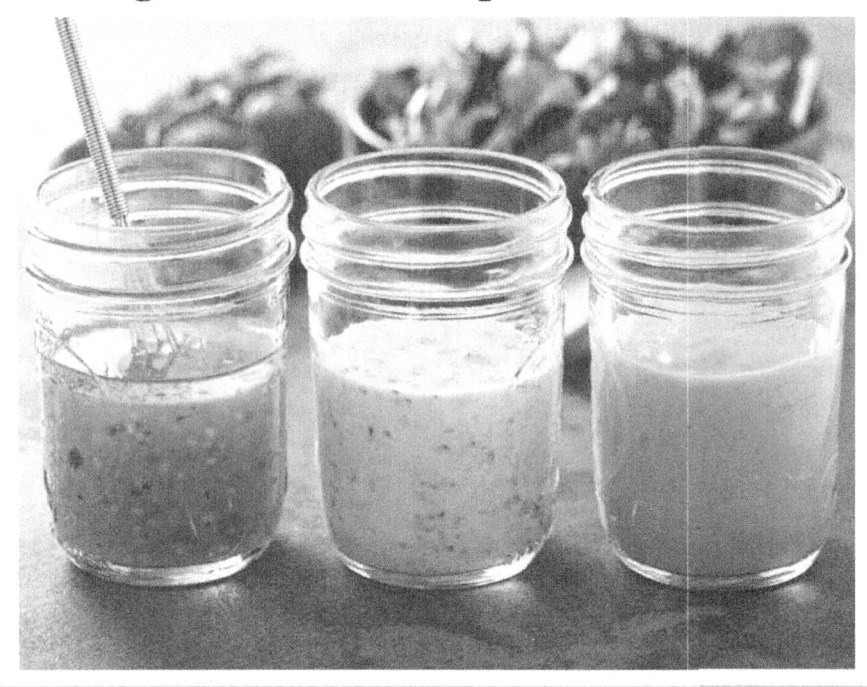

15.1 Walnut Pesto

Preparation time-10 minutes| Cook time-0 minutes| Total time-10 minutes| Servings-one cup |Difficulty-Easy

Nutritional Facts- Calories: 106; Total Fat: 11g; Total Carbs: 1g; Sugar: <1g; Fiber: <1g; Protein: 2g; Sodium: 120mg

Ingredients

- Two tablespoons of extra-virgin olive oil
- Half cup of baby spinach
- A quarter teaspoon of sea salt
- A quarter cup of walnuts
- Two minced garlic cloves
- Two tablespoons of basil leaves

Instructions

1. In a blender or food processor, combine all the ingredients.
2. Pulse for 15 to 20 (1-second) bursts or until everything is finely chopped.

15.2 Spinach Pesto

Preparation time-10 minutes| Cook time-0 minutes| Total time-10 minutes| Servings-One cup |Difficulty-Easy

Nutritional Facts- Calories: 218; Total Fat: 22g; Total Carbs: 3g; Sugar: <1g; Fiber: <1g; Protein: 6g; Sodium: 372mg

Ingredients

- Two tablespoons fresh basil leaves
- Two tablespoons of extra-virgin olive oil
- Half cup of fresh baby spinach
- Two tablespoons of pine nuts
- Two minced garlic cloves
- A quarter teaspoon of sea salt
- One ounce of grated parmesan cheese

Instructions

1. In a blender or food processor, combine all the ingredients.
2. Pulse for 15 to 20 (1-second) bursts or until everything is finely chopped.

15.3 Anti-Inflammatory Mayonnaise

Preparation time-10 minutes| Cook time-0 minutes| Total time-10 minutes| Servings-one cup| Difficulty-Easy

Nutritional Facts- Calories: 169; Total Fat: 20g; Total Carbs: <1g; Sugar: 0g; Fiber: 0g; Protein: <1g; Sodium: 36mg

Ingredients

- One tablespoon of apple cider vinegar
- One egg yolk
- Half teaspoon of Dijon mustard
- ¾ cup of extra-virgin olive oil
- Pinch sea salt

Instructions

1. Combine the cider vinegar, mustard, egg yolk, and salt in a blender or food processor.
2. Remove the top spout from the blender or food processor when it is going. Drizzle in the olive oil slowly, one drip at a time to begin. Continue to operate the processor after around 15 drops and apply the oil in a thin stream before emulsification. You may change the thickness by adjusting the volume of oil. The mayonnaise may get smoother if you apply more fat.
3. In a securely packed bottle, keep this refrigerated for up to 4 days.

15.4 Stir-Fry Sauce

Preparation time-5 minutes| Cook time-0 minutes| Total time-5 minutes| Servings-One cup |Difficulty-Easy

Nutritional Facts- Calories: 24; Total Fat: 0g; Total Carbs: 4g; Sugar: 2g; Fiber: 0g; Protein: 1g; Sodium: 887mg

Ingredients

- Two minced garlic cloves
- Two tablespoons of low-sodium soy sauce
- Juice of one lime
- Half tablespoon of arrowroot powder
- Half tablespoon of grated fresh ginger

Instructions

1. In a small bowl, whisk together all the ingredients together.

15.5 Ginger-Teriyaki Sauce

Preparation time-5 minutes| Cook time-0 minutes| Total time-5 minutes| Servings-One cup |Difficulty-Easy

Nutritional Facts- Calories: 41; Total Fat: 0g; Total Carbs: 10g; Sugar: 7g; Fiber: 0g; Protein: 1g; Sodium: 882mg

Ingredients

- Two tablespoons of pineapple juice
- Half tablespoon of grated fresh ginger
- Half teaspoon of garlic powder
- Two tablespoons of low-sodium soy sauce
- One tablespoon of packed brown sugar
- Half tablespoon of arrowroot powder or cornstarch

Instructions

1. In a small bowl, whisk all the ingredients together.
2. Keep refrigerated in a tightly sealed container for up to 5 days.

15.6 Garlic Aioli

Preparation time-5 minutes| Cook time-0 minutes| Total time-5 minutes| Servings-One cup |Difficulty-Easy

Nutritional Facts- Calories: 169; Total Fat: 20g; Total Carbs: <1g; Sugar: 0g; Fiber: 0g; Protein: <1g; Sodium: 36mg

Ingredients

- Three finely minced garlic cloves
- Half cup of anti-inflammatory mayonnaise

Instructions

1. In a small bowl, whisk the ingredients to combine.
2. Keep refrigerated in a tightly sealed container for up to 4 days.

15.7 Raspberry Vinaigrette

Preparation time-5 minutes| Cook time-0 minutes| Total time-5 minutes| Servings- One cup |Difficulty-Easy

Nutritional Facts- Calories: 167; Total Fat: 19g; Total Carbs: <1g; Sugar: 0g; Fiber: 0g; Protein: <1g; Sodium: 118mg

Ingredients

- A quarter cup of apple cider vinegar
- Three finely minced garlic cloves
- 1/8 teaspoon of freshly ground black pepper
- 3/4 cup of extra-virgin olive oil
- A quarter cup of fresh raspberries, crushed with the back of a spoon
- Half teaspoon of sea salt

Instructions

1. In a small bowl, whisk together all the ingredients.
2. Keep refrigerated in a tightly sealed container for up to 5 days.

15.8 Lemon-Ginger Vinaigrette

Preparation time-5 minutes| Cook time-0 minutes| Total time-5 minutes| Servings-One cup |Difficulty-Easy

Nutritional Facts- Calories: 167; Total Fat: 19g; Total Carbs: <1g; Sugar: 0g; Fiber: 0g; Protein: <1g; Sodium: 118mg

Ingredients

- A quarter cup of freshly squeezed lemon juice
- One minced garlic clove
- 1/8 teaspoon of freshly ground black pepper
- 3/4 cup of extra-virgin olive oil
- One tablespoon of grated fresh ginger
- Half teaspoon of sea salt

Instructions

1. In a small bowl, whisk all the ingredients.
2. Keep refrigerated in a tightly sealed container for up to 5 days.

15.9 Peanut Sauce

Preparation time-5 minutes| Cook time-0 minutes| Total time-5 minutes| Servings-One cup| Difficulty-Easy

Nutritional Facts- Calories: 143; Total Fat: 11g; Total Carbs: 8g; Sugar: 2g; Fiber: 1g; Protein: 6g; Sodium: 533mg

Ingredients

- Two tablespoons of creamy peanut butter
- Two minced garlic cloves
- Half tablespoon of freshly grated ginger
- Half cup of lite coconut milk
- Two tablespoons of freshly squeezed lime juice
- One tablespoon of low-sodium or gluten-free soy sauce or tamari

Instructions

1. In a blender or food processor, process all the ingredients until smooth.
2. Keep refrigerated in a tightly sealed container for up to 5 days.

15.10 Garlic Ranch Dressing

Preparation time-5 minutes| Cook time-0 minutes| Total time-5 minutes| Servings- one cup |Difficulty-Easy

Nutritional Facts- Calories: 17, Total Fat: 0g; Total Carbs: 3g; Sugar: 2g; Fiber: 0g; Protein: 2g; Sodium: 140mg

Ingredients

- One minced garlic clove
- Two tablespoons of chopped fresh dill
- Zest of one lemon
- 1/8 teaspoon of freshly cracked black pepper
- ¾ cup of non-fat plain Greek yogurt
- Two tablespoons of chopped fresh chives
- Half teaspoon of sea salt

Instructions

1. In a small bowl, whisk together all the ingredients.
2. Keep refrigerated in a tightly sealed container for up to 5 days.

15.11 Coconut Herb Dressing

Preparation time-5 minutes| Cook time-0 minutes| Total time-5 minutes| Servings-One cup |Difficulty-Easy

Nutritional Facts- Calories: 14; Total Fat: 1g; Total Carbohydrates: 2g; Sugar: 0g; Fiber: 1g; Protein: 0g; Sodium: 172mg

Ingredients

- Two tablespoons of freshly squeezed lemon juice
- One tablespoon of snipped fresh chives

- Pinch freshly ground black pepper
- Eight ounces plain coconut yogurt
- Two tablespoons of chopped fresh parsley
- Half teaspoon of salt

Instructions

1. In a medium bowl, whisk together all the ingredients together.
2. Refrigerate in an airtight container.

15.12 Avocado Dressing

Preparation time-10 minutes| Cook time-0 minutes| Total time-10 minutes| Servings-One cups |Difficulty-Easy

Nutritional Facts- Calories: 33; Total Fat: 3g; Total Carbohydrates: 2g; Sugar: 0g; Fiber: 1g; Protein: 0g; Sodium: 14mg

Ingredients

- Half cup of plain coconut yogurt
- Half ripe avocado
- Two tablespoons of freshly squeezed lemon juice
- Half tablespoon of chopped fresh cilantro
- Half chopped scallion

Instructions

1. In a food processor, blend all the ingredients until smooth.
2. Refrigerate in an airtight container.

15.13 Berry Vinaigrette

Preparation time-15 minutes| Cook time-0 minutes| Total time-15 minutes| Servings-one cup |Difficulty-Easy

Nutritional Facts- Calories: 73; Total Fat: 7g; Total Carbohydrates: 3g; Sugar: 2g; Fiber: 0g; Protein: 0g; Sodium: 210mg

Ingredients

- Half cup of balsamic vinegar
- Two tablespoons of freshly squeezed lemon or lime juice
- One tablespoon of lemon or lime zest
- ¾ cup of berries, fresh or frozen, no added sugar
- Three tablespoons of extra-virgin olive oil
- One tablespoon of raw honey or maple syrup
- One tablespoon of Dijon mustard

- Half teaspoon of freshly ground black pepper
- One teaspoon of salt

Instructions

1. In a blender, purée all the ingredients together until smooth.
2. Refrigerate in an airtight container for up to five days.

15.14 Almost Caesar Salad Dressing

Preparation time-10 minutes| Cook time-0 minutes| Total time-10 minutes| Servings-One cup |Difficulty-Easy

Nutritional Facts- Calories: 166; Total Fat: 19g; Total Carbohydrates: 0g; Sugar: 0g; Fiber: 0g; Protein: 0g; Sodium: 184mg

Ingredients

- Three tablespoons of apple cider vinegar
- Two minced garlic cloves
- Freshly ground black pepper
- 3/4 cup of extra-virgin olive oil
- Two anchovy fillets
- Half teaspoon of salt

Instructions

1. In a blender or food processor, purée all the ingredients until smooth.
2. Refrigerate in an airtight container and use within one week.

15.15 Cherry-Peach Chutney with Mint

Preparation time-15 minutes| Cook time-0 minutes| Total time-15 minutes| Servings-One cup |Difficulty-Easy

Nutritional Facts- Calories: 42; Total Fat: 0g; Total Carbohydrates: 10g; Sugar: 7g; Fiber: 2g; Protein: 1g; Sodium: 76mg

Ingredients

- Half diced medium red onion
- One tablespoon of freshly squeezed lemon juice
- Half teaspoon of apple cider vinegar
- Half tablespoon of chopped fresh mint leaves
- Half of one (10-ounce) bag of frozen no-added-sugar peach chunks, thawed, drained, coarsely chopped, juice reserved
- Two tablespoons of coarsely chopped dried cherries
- Half tablespoon of raw honey or maple syrup
- 1/8 teaspoon of salt

Instructions

1. In a medium mixing bowl, combine the peach chunks.
2. Combine the onion, lemon juice, cherries, cider vinegar, honey, and salt in a large mixing bowl.
3. Allow 30 minutes for the mixture to rest before serving.
4. Stir in the mint only before serving.
5. Refrigerate for no longer than three days in an airtight jar.

15.16 Rosemary-Apricot Marinade

Preparation time-15 minutes| Cook time-0 minutes| Total time-15 minutes| Servings-One cups |Difficulty-Easy

Nutritional Facts- Calories: 69; Total Fat: 6g; Total Carbohydrates: 3g; Sugar: 3g; Fiber: 0g; Protein: 0g; Sodium: 159mg

Ingredients

- Half quartered red onion
- Two tablespoons of apple cider vinegar
- One tablespoon of raw honey or maple syrup
- One teaspoon of chopped fresh rosemary
- 1/8 teaspoon of freshly ground black pepper
- Half cup of chopped apricots, fresh or frozen
- A quarter cup of extra-virgin olive oil
- One garlic clove
- Half tablespoon of Dijon mustard
- Half teaspoon of salt

Instructions

1. In a blender or food processor, combine all the ingredients. Process until smooth.
2. Refrigerate in an airtight container for up to five days.

15.17 Green Olive Tapenade

Preparation time-10 minutes| Cook time-0 minutes| Total time-10 minutes| Servings-One cup |Difficulty-Easy

Nutritional Facts- Calories: 73; Total Fat: 8g; Total Carbohydrates: 2g; Sugar: 0g; Fiber: 1g; Protein: 0g; Sodium: 201mg

Ingredients

- Two garlic cloves
- A quarter cup of freshly squeezed lemon juice
- One cup of pitted green olives
- A quarter cup of extra-virgin olive oil

- Pinch dried rosemary
- Freshly ground black pepper
- Salt

Instructions

1. In a food processor, combine all the ingredients. Process until the mixture is almost smooth; a little chunky is fine.
2. Refrigerate in an airtight container. It will keep for several weeks.

15.18 Kale Pesto

Preparation time-15 minutes| Cook time-0 minutes| Total time-15 minutes| Servings-One cup |Difficulty-Easy

Nutritional Facts- Calories: 91; Total Fat: 8g; Total Carbohydrates: 4g; Sugar: 0g; Fiber: 1g; Protein: 2g; Sodium: 299mg

Ingredients

- Half cup of toasted almonds
- Three tablespoons of freshly squeezed lemon juice
- Two teaspoons of lemon zest
- Two cups of chopped kale leave thoroughly washed and stemmed
- Two garlic cloves
- Three tablespoons of extra-virgin olive oil
- One teaspoon of salt
- A quarter teaspoon of red pepper flakes
- Half teaspoon of freshly ground black pepper

Instructions

1. In a food processor, combine all the ingredients. Process until smooth.
2. Refrigerate in an airtight container for up to one week.

15.19 Honey-Mustard-Sesame Sauce

Preparation time-10 minutes| Cook time-0 minutes| Total time-10 minutes| Servings-One cup| Difficulty-Easy

Nutritional Facts- Calories: 67; Total Fat: 1g; Total Carbohydrates: 14g; Sugar: 12g; Fiber: 1g; Protein: 1g; Sodium: 179mg

Ingredients

- Half cup of raw honey or maple syrup
- One teaspoon of toasted sesame oil
- Half cup of Dijon mustard
- One garlic clove, minced

Instructions

1. Whisk together the Dijon mustard, garlic, honey, and sesame oil in a shallow dish.
2. Place in an airtight jar and keep refrigerated.

15.20 Chia Jam

Preparation time-15 minutes| Cook time-0 minutes| Total time-15 minutes| Servings-One jar |Difficulty-Easy

Nutritional Facts- Calories: 10; Total Fat: 0g; Total Carbohydrates: 2g; Sugar: 1g; Fiber: 1g; Protein: 0g; Sodium: 0mg

Ingredients

- Half a teaspoon of vanilla extract
- A quarter-pound of ripe fresh berries
- One tablespoon of chia seeds

Instructions

1. Purée the berries and vanilla in a food processor until smooth.
2. Pulse for 10 seconds after adding the chia seeds.
3. Place the jam in a pint jar, tighten the lid, and store it in the refrigerator. Within one week, it should be consumed.

15.21 Slow-Cooker Ghee

Preparation time-5 minutes| Cook time-2 hours| Total time-2 hours and 5 minutes| Servings-One cup | Difficulty-Easy

Nutritional Facts- Calories: 102; Total Fat: 12g; Total Carbohydrates: 0g; Sugar: 0g; Fiber: 0g; Protein: 0g; Sodium: 82mg

Ingredients

- Half pound (4 sticks) of unsalted butter

Instructions

1. Add the butter to the slow cooker. Preheat the slow cooker to full and cover it.
2. A white foam forms in around 45 minutes. This foam will turn golden brown and give off a fun, nutty scent after 1 to 2 hours. The period it takes can vary depending on your slow cooker.
3. Turn off the slow cooker until the foam has turned brown.
4. Place a strainer over a wide-mouth container and line it with a triple thickness of cheesecloth.
5. Skim off as much of the brown foam as practicable with a big spoon or ladle and discard. Carefully ladle the remaining ghee into the strainer lined with cheesecloth.
6. After straining all of the ghee, discard the cheesecloth and allow the ghee to cool to room temperature before covering the jar with an airtight lid and storing it in the refrigerator. It would last three months in the refrigerator.

15.22 Coconut Cream

Preparation time-10 minutes| Cook time-0 minutes| Total time-10 minutes| Servings-One cup| Difficulty-Easy

Nutritional Facts- Calories: 71; Total Fat: 5g; Total Carbohydrates: 8g; Sugar: 7g; Fiber: 0g; Protein: 0g; Sodium: 4mg

Ingredients

- Half of one (5.4-ounce) can of full-fat coconut cream, refrigerated overnight
- Half teaspoon of vanilla extract
- Two tablespoons of maple syrup

Instructions

1. Refrigerate or ice a medium bowl and the mixer beaters for several hours or until very cold.
2. Spoon the cooled coconut cream into the cooled bowl. Pour in the maple syrup and vanilla extract on a high-speed beat with chilled beaters before soft peaks form.
3. Refrigerate before ready to use, sealed. It would only be able to maintain its highs for a few days.

15.23 Slow-Cooker Vegetable Broth

Preparation time-10 minutes| Cook time-6 hours| Total time-6 hours and 10 minutes| Servings-One cup| Difficulty-Hard

Nutritional Facts- Calories: 36; Total Fat: 0g; Total Carbohydrates: 5g; Sugar: 1g; Fiber: 1g; Protein: 1g; Sodium: 21mg

Ingredients

- One halved fennel bulb
- Half carrot, cut into 2-inch pieces
- One fresh parsley sprig
- Half leeks halved lengthwise
- One halved onion
- One garlic head halved widthwise
- One fresh rosemary sprig
- Two cups of water
- One tablespoon of apple cider vinegar

Instructions

1. Combine all the ingredients in a slow cooker. Cook for 6 hours on high.
2. Remove all solids from the broth using a fine-mesh strainer.
3. Keep the broth refrigerated or frozen in airtight pots or containers.

Conclusion

To conclude, let us sum up what we understood in this book.

When your body detects something alien, such as an invading microbe, plant pollen, or chemical, your immune system is stimulated.

Inflammation is often triggered as a result of this. Your wellbeing is protected by intermittent bouts of inflammation aimed at genuinely dangerous attackers.

However, even though you are not being attacked by a foreign invader, inflammation will persist day after day. Inflammation will then become the adversary. Cancer, coronary failure, diabetes, asthma, obesity, and Alzheimer's disease are only a few of the main illnesses that have been related to systemic inflammation.

You could be able to reduce the chances of infection by eating the right anti-inflammatory foods. If you consistently choose the wrong ones, you risk hastening the inflammatory disease mechanism.

In this book, everything regarding anti-inflammatory goods and diet is provided. Hopefully, this information will be helpful for you to understand your body and its allergies and needs.

Made in the USA
Monee, IL
05 January 2022